The Natural Foods Diet Book

The Natural Foods Diet Book

by Mary Durkin

Drawings by Ariane Reed

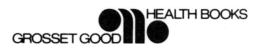
GROSSET GOOD HEALTH BOOKS

Publishers · GROSSET & DUNLAP · New York
A FILMWAYS COMPANY

Copyright © 1978 by Mary Sutro Durkin
All rights reserved
Published simultaneously in Canada
Library of Congress catalog card number: 77-93660
ISBN 0-448-14822-6

First printing
Printed in the United States of America

CONTENTS

Introduction

The Natural Foods Diet presents a new way of life. Adherents of this path will find that at the end of the rainbow lies radiant good health. Along the path, you will discover not only weight loss, but boundless energy, vitality, and a renewed enthusiasm and love of life.

Does this sound like too much to expect of any diet? Or does it excite you to think that by following a diet designed for weight control you might also discover a new way of being? The ultimate goal of the Natural Foods Diet is good health through a nutritionally balanced diet, but you will lose pounds and inches en route to that goal.

Good health means that the body, mind, and emotions are functioning at peak performance, with energy to spare. A healthy body, one that is supplied with high-quality nutritional fuel, is able to metabolize properly so that food is turned into energy rather than fat.

Most conventional diets plague the dieter with frustration, depression, and ultimately failure. We plunge into them with boundless enthusiasm and determination, spurred on by visions of a slim, trim figure, only to find ourselves weak, nervous, cranky, and exhausted at the end of a few days or weeks of dieting. Almost any diet that reduces food intake will bring about a weight loss if it is faithfully followed for a period of time. But at what price to our health? A nutritionally unbalanced diet is bound to take its toll on our entire being.

The frustrations and problems of dieting usually arise after the initial weight has been lost. We can live for only so long on just water, grapefruit, or protein. The enforced regime of dieting becomes monotonous and stressful, as the body begins to signal its need for a wider variety of nutrients. A battle rages within us: one side begging for care and nourishment, the other struggling desperately to stay on the diet.

Is this any way to live? From deep within, a voice cries "No!" and we console ourselves with an out-of-control raid on the refrigerator. As the newly lost pounds quickly creep back on, guilt—and fat—begin to reappear and we resolve to try a new crash diet. Does this pattern sound familiar? Any dieter will recognize the vicious circle that all too easily can become a life-long pattern.

Weight control cannot be maintained by any short-term diet, no matter how effective it may be at taking off pounds quickly. Because the Natural Foods Diet does not drastically reduce food intake, weight loss will be slower than it might be with a crash diet. But you will not lose your health along with the pounds. And once off, the weight should not return if natural foods have established themselves as a consistent way of life.

The Natural Foods Diet is a positive approach to weight control through a permanent change in eating patterns. It is a life-long commitment to a balanced diet of whole, "unrefined" foods. Followers of this path will soon come to realize that the Natural Foods Diet also involves a change of consciousness: a beautiful and exciting new way of thinking about food and how it affects us.

What Are Natural Foods?

Food is a gift from nature, freely offered to us for our nourishment and growth. Natural foods come to us from the earth in the purest state possible, with nothing added or taken away. They are not processed and refined, stripped of their vital nutrients, then further debilitated with chemicals and preservatives. In their original, unadulterated form, natural foods contain all the power and potential of nature herself. We can partake of this vital energy by eating these life-giving foods.

The milling of wheat into white flour provides a prime example of how refining can change a whole food into a nutritionally worthless one. When wheat is processed, its original structure is broken down as the bran and wheat germ are removed. The protein content is drastically reduced, the vitamin E is destroyed, and fifty to eighty percent of the B vitamins and valuable minerals are removed. So-called enriched bread has a minimal and incomplete amount of these nutrients restored to it, but no amount of synthetic enrichment can ever replace the loss incurred by the refining of foods.

There are billions of living cells in the body that need proper nourishment to function at their optimum level. Only the food we eat can supply the essential elements needed by the cells to regenerate, thrive, and carry out their immensely complicated and specialized activities.

These cells require a balanced and varied supply of nutrients: protein, carbohydrates, fats, vitamins, and minerals. Protein is vital for the continual maintenance and repair of muscles, bones, skin, glands, blood, and all the organs. Without protein, the cells will begin to lose their vitality and the body starts its slow trek downhill, courting fatigue, infection, and all forms of degenerative diseases.

Protein provides longer-lasting energy than carbohydrates and thus helps to keep hunger at bay. To the dieter, an adequate amount of protein intake daily is a must because protein increases the metabolic rate so calories are burned and utilized faster and more effectively.

Most nutritionists agree that we should have approximately 1 gram of protein a day for each 2 pounds of body weight. To get a quick, slightly high estimate of how much protein you need, divide your weight in half and you will come up with the minimum number of grams of protein that should be supplied by your daily diet. Meat provides protein, but it comes with a high-calorie price tag and therefore is not included in the Natural Foods Diet. Fish, chicken, eggs, tofu, soybeans, milk, cheese, yogurt, wheat germ, and sprouts are excellent sources of high-quality protein.

Carbohydrates provide quick energy for the brain, body, and muscles. In the Natural Foods Diet, carbohydrates, are supplied as natural sugars by whole grains, fruits, root vegetables, honey, and molasses. Carbohydrates are essential for good health but should only be eaten in their natural forms—and even then in moderation when on a reducing diet.

One of the most important steps you can take towards permanent weight loss is to eliminate sugar and white flour from your diet—forever. All products made from sugar and white flour are "empty foods," which have little, if any, nutritional value, and offer nothing but a high dose of calories to the body. Not only that, but these foods can lead to a low-blood-sugar syndrome. They may produce a quick surge of energy, but it soon wears off, leaving fatigue, irritability, and nervousness in its wake. The best way to satisfy a low-blood-sugar craving is not with sweets and starches, but rather by eating frequent high-protein snacks in small quantities.

Another insidious factor about these empty foods is that they lead to insatiable cravings for sweets. Have you ever experienced the miserable, sinking feeling that comes after you have plowed your way through an entire box of chocolate candy, not even conscious of what you were doing until you looked at the empty, incriminating box in your hands?

Natural foods fulfill the body's nutritional cravings and are therefore far more satisfying than high-calorie empty foods. When you are satisfied, it's easy to stop eating. For your health—and your waistline—steer clear of all foods containing sugar and white flour.

Fats are also a source of energy and are vitally important to the dieter because of their slow action and digestion. This means that the stomach feels full and hunger pangs are staved off longer after a meal that includes some fat.

A totally fat-free diet will quickly begin to show signs of its deficiency: among them are dry, brittle hair and withered, aging skin. Fats are needed in order for the body to utilize vitamins A and D, those that nourish the skin, hair, teeth, nails, and eyes. So, rather than running in the opposite direction when the word "fat" is even mentioned, think of fats and oils as part of your daily beauty treatment.

Fats should be supplied in the form of unrefined or cold-pressed liquid vegetable oils, such as safflower, sunflower, and corn oils, which contain unsaturated fatty acids. Rather than adding undesirable weight, these fatty acids are a boon to the dieter, for they stimulate the burning of stored fat. Recent tests have also shown that unsaturated fatty acids, particularly linoleic acid, actually reduce the amount of cholesterol in the blood. What good news this is to the dieter who has struggled through tasteless oil-free salad dressings for so many years. Include a few tablespoons of unsaturated vegetable oils in your daily diet: your heart, your skin, your health, and your weight will all benefit.

Hydrogenated and saturated fats—those that usually remain solid at room temperature (such as lard)—are the villains that contribute to weight gain and high cholesterol. Solid cooking fats, processed cheese, deep-fried foods, and all meats with a high fat content do not belong in the Natural Foods Diet. Margarine may be used, but be sure to buy only those brands made from unsaturated vegetable oils.

Butter may be used occasionally, though sparingly, when trying to reduce.

Vitamins, minerals, and enzymes are the microscopic substances that seem to work like magic to make the body run smoothly and efficiently. They are rarely given much attention until your system signals that your body is deficient in them. Vitamins and minerals are found abundantly in natural foods; and theoretically, all we need should be supplied by our food. Unfortunately, it is very difficult to obtain an adequate supply when following a weight-control diet with reduced food intake. Nutritional supplements, at least in the form of a multiple vitamin-mineral pill, can provide daily health insurance in this regard. Even more important than supplements, fresh raw fruits and vegetables, with their generous amount of vitamins, minerals, and enzymes, should be a mainstay of your daily diet.

Another factor of good health and weight loss is to have a certain amount of fiber or roughage in your diet every day; indeed, it is essential. Fiber, which is plentiful in raw fruits, vegetables, and bran, ensures the quick transit of food through the system.

Bran is hailed as a "wonder food" in the prevention of constipation because of its ability to absorb eight or nine times its own weight in water. When bran is added to the daily diet, foods pass more quickly through the digestive tract so there is less chance of having an uncomfortably fat, full tummy.

A few teaspoons of bran taken in a glass of tomato juice or mixed with a little yogurt before meals acts as an appetite depressant. Bran provides bulk so the stomach feels full more quickly.

Water and Salt Retention

Water retention is often a problem for dieters. As fat is burned on a reducing diet, water is actually produced in the body as a by-product of this process. Since a pound of water weighs as much as a pound of fat, the scales will not reflect a weight loss until the water is shed.

Water itself is not the culprit and cannot be blamed for weight gain. Don't shy away from drinking water, for the body needs at least six to eight glasses of water a day, part of which may be taken as herb tea.

Sodium and potassium are the two minerals directly responsible for the water control in the body. Sodium acts to retain water, potassium to eliminate it. When these two minerals are in proper balance, excess water will not be retained by the tissues.

To attain this mineral balance, eliminate all salty, processed foods from your diet. Gone are the days of blithely munching your way through a whole bag of potato chips or French fries.

Doctors have recently discovered that vitamin B_6 can be used as an equalizer to control the sodium-potassium balance—and thus regulate water retention. If your fingers or ankles feel puffy, and you suspect that the pounds reflected on your scales are from water rather than fat, consult your doctor about taking a vitamin B_6 supplement, with the entire B complex. Include lots of potassium-rich foods in your diet—citrus fruits, green leafy vegetables, watercress, parsley, bananas, green peppers, blackstrap molasses, and dried apricots.

Herbs

Herbs are a delight to cook with and are used to enhance the flavor of most foods. The judicious use of both fresh and dried herbs in cooking will lead to a lighter hand on the salt shaker. Sea salt, which is dried sea water, and herb salt, a combination of dried vegetables, herbs, sea salt, and kelp, are rich in minerals and should be used instead of commercial salt. Many of the recipes in this book call for sea salt or herb salt to taste, but even these should be used sparingly. If water retention is a problem for you, you should also eliminate soy sauce and tamari from your diet.

Diet for Health

Healthy foods and diet foods easily go hand in hand as natural partners. Every single bite of food consumed should provide a nutritional boost rather than empty calories. Whole, unrefined foods, like fresh fruits and vegetables, sprouts, whole grains, tofu, eggs, unprocessed cheese, seeds, and nuts, contain the highest proportion of nutrients per calories.

Compared to most other diets, the Natural Foods Diet can easily and happily be maintained throughout a lifetime. The simple reason why this diet is long lasting and effective is because it strengthens and builds the body. Most conventional crash diets, with their drastic restriction of foods and therefore essential nutrients, bring about a gradual weakening of your whole being and eventually lead to malnutrition. By following the Natural Foods Diet, you will begin to feel better and better, once your body has had time to adjust to whole foods and healthful eating patterns. Aside from the gradual, but definite, weight loss, you might not be immediately aware of other changes taking place within you.

Perhaps one day, after washing your hair, you might realize that it has taken on a shiny new luster and looks thick and beautiful. You might notice that your fingernails are longer and stronger than they've been in years. Your cheeks are rosy, your skin is soft and smooth . . . good health is beginning to radiate from within you. What wonderful surprises and unexpected bonuses you have to look forward to with the Natural Foods Diet.

You may also realize that for the first time in many years, each day is a happy, busy, and productive one. When you are well nourished, your food can provide you with an abundance of energy so you feel great all day long. Part of that new-found energy can be spent exercising in order to burn calories, take off inches, and redistribute weight.

Happily, the benefits of exercise do not stop there. Exercise improves muscle tone and increases the effectiveness and capacity of the lungs, heart, and circulatory system. Toxins are eliminated through sweating, and tensions are released through strenuous physical activity. When done on a regular basis, exercise can bring us closer to our goal of good health by making the entire system function more efficiently. The incentives are all there . . . now find your jogging shoes or tennis racquet.

In making a commitment to the Natural Foods Diet, we must be aware that the mental and emotional aspects of dieting are equally as important as the physical regime. As total beings, we are obviously composed of more than just our physical bodies. The mind, emotions, and even the spirit play a crucial role in successful dieting and weight control.

The mind is an incredibly powerful and complex tool that we can use to reinforce our diet. On one level, the mind can help us to understand why the Natural Foods Diet should become a way of life. Logical creatures that we are, we need proof and reassurance that the path we are following is the right one. Reading books by experts on nutrition can convince us that only natural foods lead to optimum health and therefore maintenance of a proper weight. (See Suggested Reading List.) Mental conviction and the resulting determination to pursue a goal are crucial factors in any undertaking, especially a diet.

The mind is also the key to an understanding of our eating patterns. We must examine, in depth, how, where, why, and what we eat. The easiest way to make an honest evaluation of these factors is to keep a diary, for one week, of every single bite of food and liquid taken. Don't be self-conscious about this task or vary your normal eating habits during this period of time. This evaluation is to help you—and no one else need ever see or know about it.

Immediately after eating or drinking *anything,* write down the time of day, what you ate and approximately how much, where you ate it, and why you ate it. For example, a few entries might look like this:

10:30 a.m.
   Two donuts; standing in line at grocery store; had to wait at check-out counter, and shopping made me hungry.
11:30 a.m.
   One spoonful of peanut butter; standing at kitchen counter; it looked good when making child's lunch.
11:45 a.m.
   Crusts from peanut butter and jelly sandwich, half glass of cola; standing at kitchen sink; didn't want to throw out child's unfinished lunch.

Before you even realize it, you might have eaten hundreds of calories, many of them empty ones, without even sitting down to a full meal. Keeping a journal for one week should lead to an awareness of exactly how much food you actually consume day by day.

Too often, dieters complain that they "hardly eat a thing" and still cannot lose weight. Be honest with yourself and determine whether the skimpy meals you eat at the table are only a small part of your overall daily food intake. Before eating anything, make a conscious decision to determine whether the nutritional value is worth the calories. If it's not good for you, it's not worth eating.

Meditations on the "New You"

Psychologically, the Natural Foods Diet is far easier to follow and maintain than any other reducing program because of its positive orientation. Instead of dwelling on the negative aspects usually associated with dieting— the self-discipline and deprivation—concentrate on building health through proper nutrition. When you don't feel deprived, you won't be as tempted to go on a binge. Chocolate cake and jelly donuts will begin to lose their appeal once you understand how such foods undermine your health.

Once your body has adjusted to healthful eating patterns, your cravings may even take a new line of direction. It may be that one day you can't seem to eat enough sunflower seeds or bananas. These are normal, healthy cravings, prompted by the body's search for a particular nutrient that it needs then. Become aware of these inner signals and listen to what your body is trying to tell you. You might even look up the nutritional composition of the particular food you crave and try to determine what vitamin or mineral the body is seeking. Perhaps you will need to increase your vitamin and mineral supplements for a while.

The mind can also be made to work on a deeper subconscious level to help develop a new self-image. Find a time during the day to sit quietly by yourself for a few minutes. If you meditate regularly, this would be the perfect time to practice the following exercise.

Meditating

Close your eyes and let every muscle in your body go completely limp. Concentrate on your slow, deep rhythmic breathing. If thoughts come into your head, just let them go and return your attention to your breathing. After about five minutes, or whenever you feel something like a loose rag doll, form a picture in your mind of the new you. See and feel yourself the way you would like to be: happy, healthy, and thin. Perhaps you will find yourself, clad in a brief bikini, running joyously in and out of the waves along a sandy beach. Or, dressed in bright new stretch pants, you might be skiing effortlessly down a beautiful snowy mountain.

However you picture yourself, "feel" is the key word, for *emotion* is the catalyst that acts on the subconscious to bring your ideal into being. Hold the image in your mind with determination and conviction, and never let doubt creep in. You must truly feel yourself living as the new you.

If this exercise is practiced often enough on a regular basis, the conscious mind will gradually begin to construct a pattern on the subconscious level. When the subconscious understands what it is being asked and told through constant reinforcement, it will begin to work in its mysterious, but powerful, ways to make the "outer you" conform to the "inner you."

This may sound like a simple and perhaps dubious process, but the mind is capable of performing incredible feats. If a psychosomatic illness can be triggered by the mind, why not channel this tremendous potential in a positive direction and make it work for your benefit? Try it. You will be amazed by the results.

Emotional Patterns

Emotions also have a crucial effect on eating patterns and weight control. Negative emotions, such as anger, boredom, fear, and frustration can trigger irrational eating binges, and food can become an emotional crutch. If you automatically reach into the refrigerator after an emotional crisis—and there may be many such times in the course of a single day—stop for a minute and think before you eat. Are you really hungry? Or are you angry or lonely? Perhaps a few minutes of meditation or a run around the block would bring more satisfaction than ice cream or cake.

When the nerves are properly nourished by natural foods, containing a generous supply of vitamins and minerals, emotions are far more stable. With plenty of calcium and B vitamins in your diet, you will no longer feel as if you were on an emotional seesaw all day long.

Just as the Natural Foods Diet promotes an understanding of food and its effect on the body, it also kindles a new awareness of ourselves as total beings. When we are eating foods in their purest, most natural forms, we gradually and very subtly begin to feel more in harmony with nature. We sense that the beauty and perfection of nature are not just around us, but within us. With those feelings comes a deeper understanding of what is truly meant by the words "love thyself." Natural foods not only nourish the body, but they can also open the door to spiritual growth and attunement with nature and the world around us.

Why Bother with Breakfast?

Changing to natural foods also entails rethinking your ideas about menu planning. Plan a nutritionally balanced day, rather than just organizing a meal for dinner, and letting breakfast and lunch go astray.

Breakfast is the most important meal of the day. Especially for dieters. You have the whole active day ahead of you to burn off your breakfast. Adelle Davis, the respected nutritionist, suggests that the most healthful eating pattern is to "eat breakfast like a king, lunch like a prince, and dinner like a pauper."*

The food we eat at breakfast determines our energy and blood sugar levels throughout the day. Most dieters who skip breakfast are familiar with the fatigue and irritability that creep upon them by midmorning or late afternoon. Not only must we cope with those unpleasant sensations, but we are also beseiged by an overwhelming desire to fill our empty stomachs, which are actually growling aloud in demand for food. At that moment, weak, cranky, and starving, hardly the picture of

*Adelle Davis, *Let's Eat Right to Keep Fit* (New York: Harcourt, Brace, 1970).

health, we will eat anything to fill the gnawing gap within us.

When dinnertime finally arrives, we feel we deserve a good meal to make up for the day's suffering and deprivation. Little do we realize that a huge dinner stays with us through the night and can all too easily turn to fat while we are sleeping.

If you are one of many people who claim that you are not hungry at breakfast time, try eating a smaller dinner than usual. By morning, your stomach will be empty and you should have a healthy appetite for a morning meal. Try to reestablish proper eating patterns and get your hunger channeled in the right time cycle.

Nibble Your Way through the Day

Happily for the dieter, your eating need not be confined to three meals a day. Nibbling between meals is fine and actually encouraged on the Natural Foods Diet. By spreading your food intake throughout the entire day, you will be able to keep your energy and blood-sugar levels at a constant high, so you feel good all day long.

Raw vegetables are a good snack because they can be eaten in fairly large quantities without causing a gain in weight. To make raw vegetables more appealing, prepare a day's supply ahead of time and store them in the refrigerator next to a yummy dip. Small portions of high-protein foods—seeds, nuts, or cheese—are also recommended as snacks between meals, but make sure they are really little nibbles and not mini-meals. A few nuts means four or five, not fifteen or twenty, and a little cheese means a thin slice, not a whole grilled cheese sandwich. Carry a bag of un-hulled sunflower seeds with you wherever you go. They will provide a lot of oral satisfaction because your mouth will be in constant motion, and they are almost impossible to overeat because you have to work so hard for each little bite of food.

A cup of hot or iced herb tea or a glass of fresh carrot juice can work wonders at taking the edge off your appetite. And don't forget a glass of water now and then during the day: its effects may not be long lasting, but it's good

for you and will temporarily stave off hunger pangs.

Calories Do Count

There is no need to count calories fanatically on the Natural Foods Diet, but do be aware that certain foods should be used sparingly. Use a miser's hand with mayonnaise, whipped cream, butter, and peanut butter. Even though these foods are indeed natural and delicious, they are fattening and add unwanted calories as quick as a wink. Save these treats for the days when you feel especially thin.

It's easy to substitute less fattening ingredients for high-calorie ones. A salad dressing or vegetable dip made from one cup of mayonnaise contains more than 1,600 calories, as compared to one made of yogurt, with 150 calories. With weight loss in mind, the choice between the two should not be a difficult one to make. Go ahead and have a baked potato, but fill it with yogurt and chives, instead of butter and sour cream. Learn to enjoy whole grain toast spread with cinnamon apple butter or homemade strawberry jam—it's so delicious you won't even miss the butter. When every bite counts, little things can mean a lot.

Food Is Beautiful

Food presentation is always important, but especially to the dieter. When food is beautifully displayed, less attention is drawn to the actual size of the portion. To make a small amount of food seem larger than it is, serve the meal on large plates and garnish them lavishly. A main course can be visually and nutritionally enhanced by generous sprigs of watercress or parsley, carrot curls, green pepper rings, radish roses or small bunches of alfalfa sprouts. There is a world of difference in the appeal of a chicken that is plopped on a platter all by itself and one that is nestled amidst a bed of parsley. Fresh fruit becomes an elegant dessert when served on shiny green leaves and sprinkled with glistening rose petals or violets. The small touch of a decorative garnish can transform the ordinary into a sensational meal.

Weight Loss Vs. Weight Maintenance

One of the big plusses about the Natural Foods Diet is that you don't have to plan separate meals each day—one for you and one for the nondieters in your household. Because the Natural Foods Diet is designed to promote good health, not just weight loss, your entire family will reap lifelong benefits when you make the change to wholesome, unrefined foods. Make the transition to natural foods gradually, without any dramatic pronouncements. Your family is probably quite satisfied with their accustomed diet, and they needn't know, at least at first, what exciting changes lie in their future.

The key difference between *weight loss* and *weight maintenance* is the size of the portions consumed. Only the quantities, not the food itself, change while reducing. You don't have to eat like a bird, but do use moderation and control. No matter how healthy the food may be, you will not lose weight if you overeat.

Take small servings at mealtime. Savor and enjoy each bite. The portions will actually seem larger and more satisfying if you chew your food thoroughly, instead of gulping it down. Thorough chewing will also ensure proper digestion and assimilation of food.

Always stop eating when you are full. There is no rule, no matter what we were taught as children, that you have to finish every bite on your plate. For some people, this idea takes quite a conscious effort to undo. Nor is there any reason to finish scraps off your children's plates as you wash the dishes. Feed the scraps to the dog, or save them for the compost pile. Better there than in you.

Menu Planning

Be flexible when planning meals. Variety is important on any diet, and the Natural Foods Diet offers tremendous possibilities for creativity and personal preferences. Be aware that your daily food intake should include protein, carbohydrates, fats, vitamins, and minerals, but these should not all be piled into a huge evening meal. For optimum health, raw foods should be included as a part of every meal.

The following list offers some suggestions for menu planning by the seasons. Remember, have small servings of everything. Recipes for starred items are included in the following section.

Summer:

Breakfast	Yogurt sundae*
	Herb tea
Snack	Fresh fruit cocktail*
Lunch	Salade Niçoise*
	2 Lemon Crisps*
	Low-fat milk
Snack	Pickled Vegetable Antipasto*
Dinner	Green Herb Gazpacho*
	Vegetarian Bleu Cheese Delight*
	½ cup Strawberry Ice*
	Herb tea

Fall:

Breakfast	Dutch Apple Oatmeal*
	Herb tea
Snack	1 small banana
Lunch	Spanish Omelet*
	Tossed green salad with sprouts
	½ cup yogurt or low-fat milk
Snack	1 cup Carrot Juice*
Dinner	Hearty Vegetable Soup*
	Molded Herb Cheese*
	½ toasted pita bread
	Herb tea

Winter:

Breakfast	½ grapefruit
	1 egg, cooked your favorite way
	1 Bran muffin* with Strawberry Jam*
	Herb tea
Snack	Small handful of sunflower seeds
Lunch	Curried Zucchini Soup*
	½ pita bread with 1 ounce melted cheese and sprouts
	Low-fat milk
Snack	Raw Vegies and Green Goddess Dip*
Dinner	Fillet of Sole Bonne Femme*
	⅓ cup brown rice
	Celery Root Remoulade*
	Yogurt Fruit Parfait*
	Herb tea

Spring:

Breakfast	Cottage Cheese Pancakes*
	Blueberry Sauce*
	Herb tea
Snack	5–6 almonds
Lunch	1 cup Quick Tomato Herb Soup*
	1 Norwegian flatbread
	1 ounce Cheddar cheese
	1 apple
	Iced herb tea
Snack	½ cup yogurt with 2 tsp bran
Dinner	Curried Soy Beans*
	Spinach and Sprout Salad*
	Strawberry Delight*
	Herb tea

Where to Find Natural Foods

As more and more people express their concern with health and nutrition, natural foods are becoming more readily accessible. The "health food" stores have always carried unrefined products; but now, even supermarkets, in response to consumers' demands, are beginning to stock natural foods. There are still a few items (many are listed in the Glossary) that can usually be purchased only at health food stores. But natural foods are the wave of the future, and it is up to each one of us to ask our local stores to stock a wider variety of unrefined products.

"Organic food," whether it be fruits, vegetables, nuts, seeds, or chickens, is raised without the use of chemical fertilizers, pesticides, hormones, antibiotics, or other man-made products. If you can find a reliable source of organic foods, buy your supplies there. If not, do the best you can, knowing that every step you take towards a natural diet is an important one.

Become a "label reader." Every time you reach for a can or package, check out all the ingredients. Chances are good that if you can't even pronounce the words on the label, you don't want to eat that particular food; for it probably contains chemicals that could be harmful to your health. This may seem like a big chore at first, but you will soon come to know instinctively which foods are wholesome and life giving and which ones should remain on the shelf.

So Much to Gain

There are many people who are genuinely concerned with health and nutrition but are afraid that natural foods will put too large a dent in their food budgets. Actually, wholesome foods are no more expensive than junk foods because you get far greater food value for your dollars. And hopefully, as improved nutrition reflects itself in better health, you will receive an unexpected bonus: money in your pocket, which need not be spent on doctors' bills. Eating a diet of natural foods is one of the best steps you can take towards preventive medicine, because the body has an amazing ability to heal and protect itself if supplied with the proper nutrients.

The Natural Foods Diet provides all the essential elements needed so we can function at our optimum level and truly live life to its fullest. The goal is an ideal one, but well worth striving for. When we live in the peak of health, life itself becomes more meaningful as we find peace within ourselves and a sense of harmony and attunement with nature and our world.

You may have pounds to lose, but there is so much good health to gain and a beautiful, exciting life to live. Don't you owe it to yourself to give the Natural Foods Diet a wholehearted try?

Note: Some ingredients in the recipes may be unfamiliar to you. In the back of the book is a Glossary of Natural Ingredients, which will define these foods.

1
Little Nibbles and Drinks

A word about canning: In this chapter and in others in the book, there are recipes that call for doing your own canning. Especially for a natural foods diet, there is nothing more enjoyable than your own canned foods. They are completely natural; absent are extraneous chemicals—and you know exactly what the contents are. However, canning, if done improperly, can lead to botulism, which can be fatal. So great care must be exercised in canning all foods. This is especially so with nonacid foods where the development of *Clostridium botulinum* can occur. Consult a cookbook that has detailed instructions on the canning process; or buy a book on canning. Also, canning kits come complete with the manufacturer's instructions on the method.

In any case, if canning is done correctly, you need not worry about the foods spoiling.

Pickled Vegetable Antipasto

Make a big batch of these crunchy sweet-and-sour vegetables ahead of time, to have on hand whenever you need a quick snack or appetizer. The list of ingredients may be a long one, but these are delicious and easy to make.

6 carrots, peeled and cut in thin 1½-inch sticks
18 tiny white onions, peeled
1 small cauliflower, cut into florets
1 small bunch broccoli, cut into florets
5 celery stalks, peeled and cut in thin 1½-inch sticks
2 zucchini, cut in thin strips
1 green pepper, seeded and cut in thin strips
2 red peppers, seeded and cut in thin strips

6 cups water
2½ cups white wine vinegar
⅔ cup honey
2 tbs mustard seed
3 bay leaves, broken up
1 tsp celery seed
1 tsp dill seed
8 whole peppercorns
4 whole cloves
1 tbs herb salt
3 garlic cloves, peeled
cayenne

Cut vegetables into specified sizes. Place water, vinegar, honey, mustard seed, bay leaves, celery seed, dill seed, peppercorns, cloves, and herb salt in a large saucepan. Bring mixture to a boil. Reduce heat, cover, and simmer for 15 minutes. Add carrots, onions, cauliflower, and broccoli to the pot. Bring to a boil and cook for 30 seconds. Add zucchini, celery, and red and green peppers. Turn off heat and let stand for 30 seconds. Strain vegetables and return liquid to pot. Bring to a boil again.

Place 1 garlic clove and a pinch of cayenne in each of three hot sterilized quart canning jars. Tightly pack vegetables into jars, alternating the different vegetables. Pour boiling liquid into jars, leaving ½-inch head space. Run a knife down the inside of each jar to get out any air bubbles. Seal at once. Let stand in a cool, dark cupboard for 2 weeks, for the best flavor. If you're in a hurry, wait at least 24 hours. Refrigerate after opening. Makes 3 quarts.

Cauliflower à la Grecque

⅔ cup white wine vinegar
1 cup white wine
1 tsp honey
2 slices lemon
6 parsley sprigs
8 peppercorns
1 tsp pickling spice
herb salt to taste
1 cauliflower, cut in florets
1 green pepper, seeded and cut in thin strips
1 sweet red pepper, seeded and cut in thin strips
½ cup black pitted olives
2 tbs chopped parsley
2 tbs chopped scallions

Place vinegar, white wine, honey, lemon, parsley sprigs, peppercorns, pickling spice, and herb salt in a saucepan and bring to a boil. Simmer for 15 minutes. Strain and return liquid to pan. Bring liquid to a boil and add cauliflower. Cover and simmer 6 to 7 minutes, until cauliflower is barely tender. Add green and red pepper strips the last 30 seconds of cooking. Pour mixture into a bowl and stir in olives, chopped parsley and scallions. When

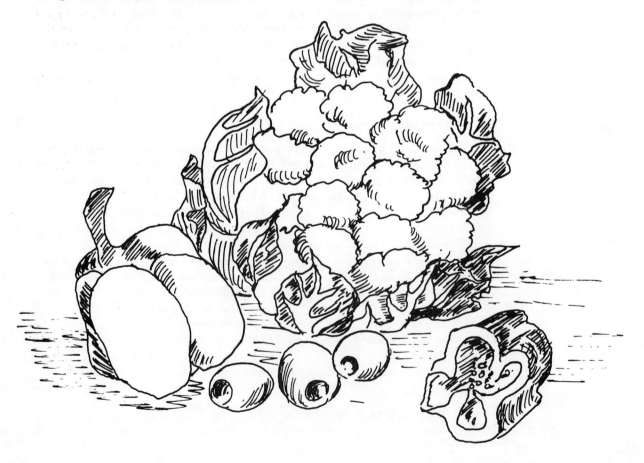

cool, cover, and refrigerate at least 12 hours. Drain well before serving. Flavor improves on standing. Makes 1 quart.

Variation: Add 10 to 12 cherry tomatoes when the liquid has cooled for a lovely color combination.

Dilly Beans

2½ cups water	8 sprigs fresh dill
2½ cups white wine vinegar	cayenne
1 tbs herb salt	2 pounds fresh green beans
4 cloves garlic, peeled	

Place water, vinegar, and herb salt in a saucepan and bring to a boil. Place 1 garlic clove, 2 dill sprigs, and a pinch of cayenne in each of 4 sterilized pint-size canning jars. Snap ends off beans and pack tightly into jars. Pour boiling liquid into jars, leaving ½-inch head space. Run a knife around the insides of the jars to get out air bubbles. Seal tightly with lids and submerge jars in a pot filled with boiling water. Boil for 10 minutes in the water bath. Remove and cool. Store jars in a cool, dark cupboard until needed. Makes 4 pints.

Marinated Mushrooms

½ cup water	1 tsp herb salt
½ cup tarragon vinegar	1 lb small fresh mushrooms
½ tsp dill seeds	3 tbs chopped parsley
1 bay leaf	3 tbs chopped scallions
6 peppercorns	
4 whole cloves	
1 1-inch piece cinnamon	

Place water, vinegar, dill seeds, bay leaf, peppercorns, cloves, cinnamon, and herb salt in a saucepan. Simmer, covered, for 15 minutes. Wash mushrooms and cut off the ends of the stems. Mix mushrooms with parsley and scallions. Pack tightly into a 1-quart canning jar. Pour hot liquid over mushrooms. Place lid on jar and refrigerate for 12 hours.
Serves 6.

Eggplant Caviar

1 eggplant	2 tbs chopped parsley
1 tbs safflower oil	2 tbs chopped
1 garlic clove, minced	scallions
1 onion, chopped	herb salt and pepper
2 tomatoes, chopped	to taste
2 tsp lemon juice	

Bake whole eggplant in a 350 degree oven for 50 minutes, or until soft. Remove from oven and let cool. Then peel and chop eggplant into small pieces. Heat oil in a skillet. Sauté garlic and onion until soft. Mix all ingredients together, pour into a bowl, cover, and refrigerate until well chilled. Serve in a bowl, surrounded by small, crisp romaine lettuce leaves and/or lightly toasted pita bread.
Serves 6.

"Rabbit Food"

Raw vegetables (or "vegies," as enthusiasts often call them) are a dieter's delight, but unfortunately the high-calorie dips they are dunked in are often our undoing. This problem is easily solved by substituting yogurt for all or part of the sour cream, cream cheese, and mayonnaise usually called for.

If you have always thought that rabbit food meant only carrot and celery sticks, just wait and see what taste treats and surprises are in store for you. Try any of the following raw vegetables, choosing the peak of the seasonal crop.

Asparagus—break off tough lower stem
Beans, green or yellow—snap off stems
Beets—peel, cut into thin strips
Broccoli—break into florets
Cabbage, red and green—cut into small chunks
Carrots—you know how to fix these
Cauliflower—break into florets
Celery—string and cut into sticks
Celery root—peel, cut into thin sticks, sprinkle with lemon juice to prevent discoloring
Cherry tomatoes—leave whole
Cucumber—peel only if waxed, cut into sticks
Endive, Belgian—cut off stem end, pull leaves apart
Jerusalem artichoke—slice thin
Mushrooms—leave whole, cut off end of stem

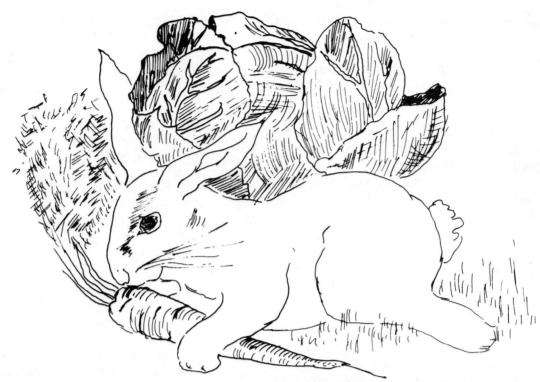

Parsley—cut into sprigs
Parsnips—cut into sticks
Peppers, red and green—seed and cut into
  strips
Radishes—cut into roses
Scallions—remove stringy ends
Snow peas—remove stem end and string
Turnips—peel and slice thin
Watercress—cut into sprigs
Zucchini—cut into sticks

Avocados

Don't shy away from the scrumptious avocado, with the mistaken idea that it adds instant pounds to your weight. The avocado is one of nature's most perfect foods and contains a heaping amount of protein, vitamins, especially E, minerals, including potassium, and unsaturated fats (these are the good ones that are easily burned by the body).

Avocado Dip

1 large avocado,   2 tsp lemon juice
  peeled and pitted   ¾ cup plain yogurt
3 scallions, minced   herb salt to taste

1 tomato, peeled,   pinch of cayenne
  chopped, and
  drained
1 to 2 mild or hot
  canned green
  chilies, chopped

Place avocado in a bowl and mash with a fork. Mix in scallions, tomato, chili peppers, and lemon juice. Gently stir in yogurt, herb salt, and cayenne. Cover tightly and refrigerate until chilled. If the top darkens, give it a good stir before serving. Serve with lots of raw vegetables.
Serves 6 to 8.

Curried Crab Dip

1 pad of tofu   pinch of cayenne
1 cup plain yogurt   herb salt to taste
1 tbs lemon juice   2 tbs chopped parsley
1 tsp to 1 tbs curry   1 7½-ounce can crab
  powder to taste   meat, flaked
2 tbs onion, minced
pinch of powdered
  ginger

Place tofu, ½ cup yogurt, lemon juice, curry powder, onion, ginger, cayenne, and herb salt in blender. Blend until smooth. Stop the blender and scrape down sides if necessary. Pour mixture into a bowl and stir in remaining ½ cup yogurt and parsley. Cover tightly and refrigerate for at least 2 hours. Stir in crab meat right before serving. Serve with raw vegetables.

Note: For a quick, spur-of-the-moment dip, stir curry powder, to taste, into yogurt.

Serves 6.

Green Goddess Dip

1 pad of tofu	¾ cup watercress
1 cup plain yogurt	leaves
1 tbs tarragon vinegar	6 scallions, chopped
1 tsp lemon juice	1 garlic clove
1 tbs anchovy paste,	pinch of cayenne
optional	herb salt to taste
¾ cup parsley,	
chopped	

Place all ingredients, except ½ cup of yogurt, in the blender. Blend until very smooth. Scrape down sides of blender if necessary. Pour into a bowl and stir in remaining ½ cup of yogurt. Cover tightly and refrigerate 4 hours. Stir gently before serving. Serve with raw vegetables.

Serves 6.

Yogurt Herb Dip

1 cup plain yogurt	2 tbs chives, minced
1 garlic clove, pressed	1–2 tsp dill
3 tbs chopped	pinch of cayenne
parsley	herb salt to taste
4 scallions, minced	¼ tsp dry mustard

Gently stir all ingredients together. Cover and refrigerate for 1 hour or overnight. Serve with raw vegetables.

This dip can serve as the basis for many variations. Experiment by adding one of the following: curry powder to taste; 2 ounces mashed bleu cheese; ½ cup finely chopped mushrooms; Dijon mustard to taste; ¼ cup chili sauce; ½ cup well-drained minced clams; 1 grated drained cucumber or 3 tbs fine-chopped walnuts.

Serves 6.

Stuffed Celery with Bleu Cheese

1 cup low-fat cottage	dash of cayenne
cheese	sea salt to taste
2 ounces bleu cheese	celery stalks, washed
1 tbs minced scallions	and peeled
1½ tbs chopped	paprika
parsley	tiny parsley sprigs

Place cottage cheese, bleu cheese, scallions, chopped parsley, cayenne, and sea salt in a small bowl. Mash with a fork until mixture is very smooth. Spread mixture in whole celery stalks; place on a plate, cover, and refrigerate for 2 hours. When well chilled, slice celery into 2-inch pieces. Sprinkle each with paprika and top with a sprig of parsley.

Stuffed Mushrooms: Prepare mixture as directed above, but stir in ⅓ cup fine-chopped mushrooms. Stuff whole mushroom caps with mixture and refrigerate until well chilled.

Serves 4.

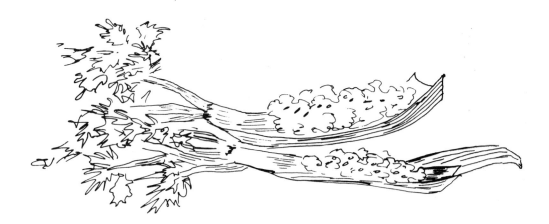

Stuffed Cherry Tomatoes

1½ cups low-fat
  cottage cheese
3 scallions, minced
3 tbs chopped parsley
2 tbs chopped chives
½ cucumber, peeled,
  seeded, chopped,
  and drained

¼ cup plain yogurt
½ tsp basil
pinch of cayenne
herb salt to taste
1 pint cherry tomatoes,
  stems removed

Mix together all ingredients except the tomatoes. Cut tops off tomatoes and use a small spoon to scoop out the pulp. (Reserve insides for another use, such as for gazpacho.) Turn tomatoes upside down to drain. Fill tomatoes with cottage cheese mixture and refrigerate for 1 hour. Arrange tomatoes on a platter, garnished liberally with parsley or watercress sprigs.
  Serves 8.

Onion Cheese Puffs

4 oz. farmer's cheese
1 tbs Parmesan cheese
1 tbs mayonnaise
2½ tbs buttermilk
2 tbs minced onion
1 tbs. chopped
  parsley

1 tsp dill
pinch of cayenne
herb salt to taste
whole wheat or rye
  Melba rounds
paprika
tiny parsley sprigs

Place first 9 ingredients in a bowl. Mash together with a fork until mixture is smooth. Spread on Melba crackers and place on a cookie sheet. Sprinkle each with a little paprika. Place on a low rack in the oven and broil until cheese is puffy and lightly browned. Garnish each with a sprig of parsley and serve hot.
  Serves 4.

Molded Herb Cheese

1 tbs unflavored
  gelatin
¼ cup cold water
¼ cup boiling water
1½ cups low-fat
  cottage cheese
½ cup buttermilk

1 garlic clove
2 tbs parsley
3 tbs chives
1 tsp thyme
1 tsp dry mustard
pinch of cayenne
herb salt to taste

Soften gelatin in cold water. Add boiling water and stir until gelatin is dissolved. Place gelatin and all remaining ingredients in blender and blend until very smooth. Pour mixture into a cold wet mold and refrigerate until set. Unmold onto a platter and surround with watercress sprigs and radish roses. Serve with toasted pita bread, thin whole wheat crackers, or Norwegian flatbread (this has the lowest calories of all).
  Serves 8.

Pickled Shrimp

2 lb shrimp, cooked
  and peeled
2 cups white wine
  vinegar
4 tbs pickling spice
1 tbs peppercorns
1 tbs honey
1 tsp dried mustard
1 tsp fresh ginger,
  minced or ¼ tsp
  powdered ginger

herb salt to taste
1 lemon, sliced
1 red onion, sliced
2 bay leaves
½ cup safflower oil
½ cup chicken broth
¼ cup parsley sprigs

Place vinegar, pickling spice, peppercorns, honey, mustard, ginger, and herb salt in a saucepan and bring to a boil. Simmer mixture for 15 minutes. Cool liquid, then strain. Mix liquid with shrimp and all remaining ingredients. Cover tightly and refrigerate for 24 hours. Drain well. Arrange shrimp on a bed of lettuce leaves and use toothpicks to spear the shrimp.
  Serves 8.

Chicken Saté

2 whole chicken
  breasts, skinned
  and boned
1 cup soy sauce
½ cup white wine
1 garlic clove, minced
1 tsp fresh ginger,
  minced

1 tbs honey
1 can water chestnuts
1 can unsweetened
  pineapple chunks
6-inch long bamboo
  skewers

Cut chicken into 1-inch cubes. Mix together the soy sauce, white wine, garlic, ginger, and honey. Marinate chicken in the mixture for at least 2 hours. Thread chicken on small bamboo skewers, alternating chicken with water chestnuts and pineapple chunks. Cook over a hot grill; or broil 5 minutes on each side. Serve warm.
  Variation: Substitute peeled shrimp or scallops for the chicken.
  Serves 4.

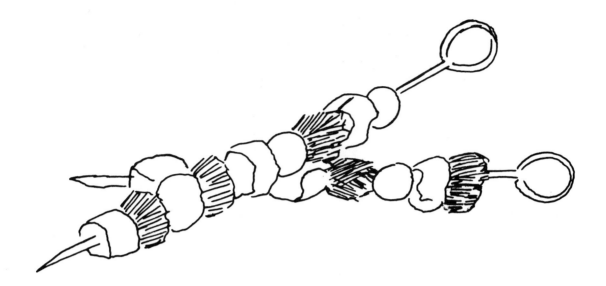

Vegetable Cocktails

Have you ever tasted a glass of sweet, freshly made carrot juice? It's pure heaven. It is low in calories, chock full of vitamins, minerals, and enzymes and ever so satisfying. One of the best investments you can make in your own health is to purchase a juicer and make juicing a daily ritual.

Carrots make the sweetest, most delicious juice of all, but don't stop there. Try mixing them with celery, parsley, beets, cabbage, spinach, or green beans. Come up with your own favorite combinations for this fabulous vitamin cocktail.

Carrot Juice

1 lb fresh carrots

Scrub carrots with a stiff brush and cut off ends. Put through a juicer and drink at once.

Vegetable Cocktail

1 cup V8 juice	2–3 drops Tabasco
juice of ½ lemon	pinch of celery seed
1 tsp Bronner's Broth	pinch of herb salt

Mix all ingredients together and pour into a tall glass over ice. If desired, serve with a cucumber or celery stick stirrer.
Serves 1.

Tomato-Yogurt Cocktail

4 cups tomato juice or V8 juice	herb salt to taste
	1 tsp Bronner's Broth
½ cup plain yogurt	dash of Tabasco
1 tsp horseradish	¼ tsp dill
2 tsp lemon juice	

Place all ingredients in blender and blend well. Serve in tall glasses over crushed ice. Sprinkle with additional dill, if desired. If you have fresh dill, that's even better.
Serves 4.

Fresh Fruit Cocktail

1 slice melon	6 strawberries
1 slice fresh pineapple	5 to 6 ice cubes

Cut fruit into small pieces and place in blender. With motor running, drop ice cubes, one at a time, into blender. Blend until smooth and fluffy. Pour into a glass and drink at once.

Note: There are endless possible variations of this drink. Experiment by mixing any of your favorite fruits together.
Serves 1.

Tutti-Frutti Grape Sangria

2 oranges	2 tbs honey
1 lemon	32 fl oz (1 qt) white
1 lime	grape juice

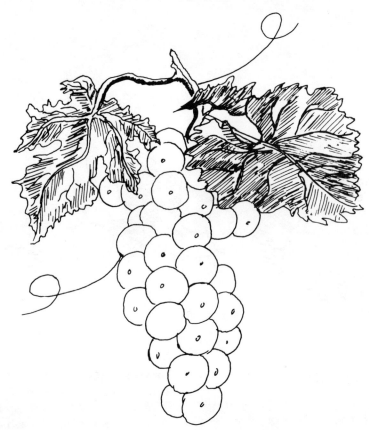

¾ cup seedless green grapes   2 cups Perrier water

Thin-slice the oranges, lemon, and lime. Place sliced fruit in a bowl and add grapes and honey. Mix well and let stand 2 hours. Add grape juice and pour into a pitcher. Refrigerate until ready to serve. Stir in Perrier water. Pour into tall glasses over ice, serving some of the fruit in each glass.

Serves 6.

Wine

There is no need to give up the pleasure and enjoyment of an occasional predinner cocktail, but do switch from alcohol to wine. Hard liquor is a nutritionally empty food, with no redeeming values (in spite of what you may think). It plays havoc with the blood-sugar level in the body, destroys vitamins, and adds hundreds of undesirable calories. But an occasional glass of wine is an entirely different matter.

Dr. Salvatore P. Lucia, professor of medicine at the University of California Medical School, has stated that wine "is a most complex biologic fluid possessing definite physiologic values. It has nutritional value due to its content of B vitamins and minerals—potassium, magnesium, sodium, calcium, iron, and phosphorus. . . . Wine helps the digestion, and its tranquilizing and sedative effects are good for the heart, arteries, blood pressure, and strengthening the walls of the capillary veins."[*] So go ahead and enjoy your wine, but remember, all things in moderation.

White Wine Spritzer
dry white wine   Perrier water

For each serving, place 2 ounces white wine in a glass filled with ice. Fill with Perrier water and serve.

Cranberry Spritzer
2 cups fresh cranberries   honey to taste
6 cups water   white wine

Place cranberries and water in a saucepan and bring to a boil. Cover and simmer for 20

[*]Linda Clark, *Get Well Naturally* (New York: Arco Publishing Co., 1974), p. 144.

minutes, or until cranberries are very soft. Pour into blender, in batches, and blend well. Strain through a fine sieve. Sweeten with honey to taste. (Use the honey judiciously as this should be a rather tart drink.) Pour into a bottle and refrigerate until needed. If you prefer not to mix it with wine, it is delicious served all by itself over ice.

To make the spritzer, fill tall glasses with ice. Pour equal parts cranberry juice and white wine into the glasses and stir well. A dash of Perrier water may be added for a little sparkle.

Serves 6 to 8.

Fat-Free, NO-Calorie Cocktail

What is the miraculous ingredient? Water! Serve water in a tall glass over crushed ice and garnish the glass with a slice of lemon or lime. For a delightful change, try sparkling Perrier water over ice.

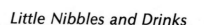

2
Super Soups

When making homemade broth for soup, remember that the richer the stock, the tastier the soup will be. There is nothing difficult or time-consuming about making broth—simply throw a few nutritious ingredients into a kettle with some water and let the broth simmer on the back of the stove for several hours. The resulting broth will be full of vitamins and minerals and, once you skim off the fat, very low in calories.

Prepare a large pot of broth when you have the time and freeze it in eight-ounce containers. It will be ready and waiting whenever the urge to make soup comes upon you and you need a quick base.

Chicken Broth

3 lb chicken pieces (carcasses, necks, wings, backs) Save extra pieces of chicken in the freezer until you have collected enough to make broth.
3 carrots, sliced
3 celery stalks, sliced
1 onion, sliced
2 leeks, sliced

8 parsley sprigs
½ tsp thyme
2 bay leaves
6 black peppercorns
2 whole cloves
1 tsp herb salt, or to taste
1 cup dry white wine, optional
3 qt water
1 tbs Bronner's Broth

Place all ingredients in a large soup pot. Bring to a boil. Reduce heat, cover, and simmer for 2½ hours. While cooking, skim off scum occasionally as it rises to the surface. Strain broth through a fine sieve or several layers of cheese-

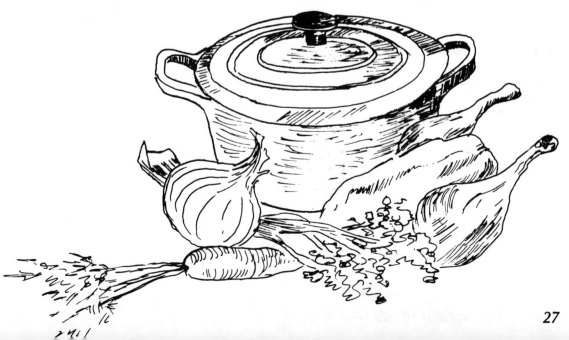

cloth. Pour into a large bowl, uncovered, and refrigerate overnight. Remove fat that rises to the surface. Use at once, or bottle it, covered, and refrigerate or freeze.

Note: the broth will keep well in the refrigerator for 3 or 4 days; if kept refrigerated longer, boil it every 3 or 4 days to prevent spoilage. Otherwise, freeze it.

Makes 2½ quarts.

Vegetable Broth

3 tbs butter	1 tsp savory
4 carrots, sliced	1 tsp herb salt
4 scallions, sliced	6 peppercorns
2 onions, chopped	2 whole cloves
4 celery stalks, sliced	1 tbs Bronner's Broth
1 turnip, sliced	1 cup dry white
3 leeks, sliced	wine, optional
8 parsley sprigs	2 qt water
2 bay leaves	

Melt butter in a large soup pot and sauté vegetables for 3 minutes. Add all remaining ingredients to pot. Bring to a boil. Reduce heat, cover, and simmer for 2 hours. Strain through a fine sieve or several layers of cheesecloth. Pour into a large bowl and refrigerate overnight in the prescribed manner. In the morning, skim off the fat that rises to the surface. Use at once, refrigerate, or freeze.

To enrich the stock nutritionally, save the cooking liquid leftover from steaming vegetables in a small jar in the refrigerator. Leftover peelings and parings from raw vegetables may also be saved in a plastic bag. When ready to make broth, add the liquid and/or peelings to the pot before simmering. Makes 1½ quarts.

Borscht with Cabbage

1 tbs. safflower oil	1 bay leaf
1 onion, chopped	¼ cup white wine,
3 cups chicken or	optional
vegetable broth	herb salt and pepper
1 bunch beets,	to taste
cooked, peeled,	⅔ cup plain yogurt
and cut into	2 tbs fresh dill,
match-sticks	chopped *or* 1 tsp

1 cup cabbage,	dried dill
shredded	

Heat oil in a saucepan and sauté onion until soft. Place onions, 1 cup broth, and one-quarter of the beets in blender. Blend until smooth. Pour mixture into saucepan and add remaining broth, beets, cabbage, bay leaf, wine, herb salt, and pepper. Cover and simmer for 10–15 minutes. Ladle into soup bowls and garnish each serving with a generous spoonful of yogurt and a sprinkling of dill.

Serves 4.

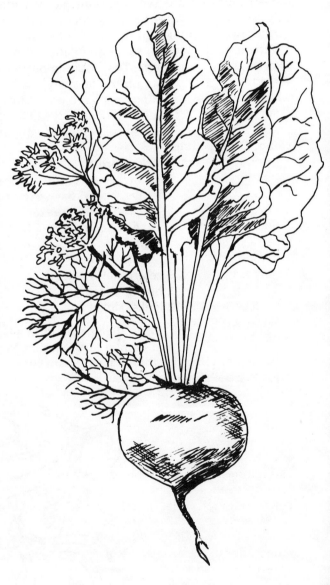

Carrot Soup à l'Orange

1 onion, chopped	herb salt to taste
1 celery stalk, chopped	pinch of cayenne
1 pound carrots, sliced	2 tsp grated orange rind
3½ cups chicken or vegetable broth	½ cup plain yogurt
	1½ tbs chopped chives

Place onion, celery, carrots, and broth in a saucepan. Bring to a boil. Reduce heat, cover, and simmer 20 minutes. Stir in herb salt, cayenne, and orange rind. Purée in blender, a few cups at a time, until very smooth. Refrigerate until well chilled or return to saucepan and reheat. Right before serving, whether hot or cold, stir in yogurt. Ladle soup into bowls and garnish with a sprinkling of chopped chives.

Variation: To add protein, and very few calories, puree 1 pad of tofu with the soup. If served hot, soup may be garnished with whole wheat croutons.

Serves 4.

Good, Old-Fashioned Chicken Soup

1 3-pound chicken, quartered	½ cup brown rice
1 onion, sliced	2 carrots, sliced ¼-inch thick
1 carrot, sliced	2 celery stalks, sliced ¼-inch thick
2 celery stalks, sliced	½ pound mushrooms, sliced thick
6 parsley sprigs	½ cup dry white wine
1 bay leaf	herb salt and pepper to taste
1 tsp basil	2 tbs chopped parsley
1 tsp thyme	
1 tbs Bronner's Broth	
6 black peppercorns	
water to cover	

Place first 11 ingredients in a large soup pot. Bring to a boil. Reduce heat, cover, and simmer for 1½ hours. Strain broth through a fine sieve or several layers of cheesecloth. Discard cooked vegetables and set aside chicken quarters. Cool broth, then skim off fat that rises to the surface. Skin and bone the chicken and cut meat into small pieces. Set aside. Return broth to soup pot and add rice, carrots, celery, herb salt and pepper. Simmer, covered, for 40 minutes. Add reserved chicken, mushrooms, and white wine. Cook 10 minutes longer. Stir in parsley right before serving.

Serves 6.

Chinese Vegetable and Tofu Soup

4 dried Chinese black mushrooms	1 cup bean sprouts
6 cups chicken broth	2 tbs sherry
½ pound snow peas, cut in half if large	2 tbs soy sauce
½ lb mushrooms, sliced	1½ tbs cornstarch
6 water chestnuts, sliced	3 scallions, minced
1½ pads tofu, cut in thin strips	dash of dark sesame oil, optional
1 cup spinach, tightly packed, stems removed, torn in small pieces	dash of white pepper

Soak dried mushrooms in water to cover for 30 minutes. Drain and squeeze dry. Remove hard stems and slice mushrooms thin. Place chicken broth in a soup pot and bring to a boil. Add dried mushrooms and snow peas. Simmer for 3 minutes. Add fresh mushrooms, water chestnuts, and tofu. Simmer for 3 minutes. Add spinach and bean sprouts. Mix sherry and soy sauce with the cornstarch. Add to soup and stir until slightly thickened. Stir in scallions, sesame oil, and white pepper. Serve at once.

To increase the protein value of the soup, add two slightly beaten eggs. Remove finished soup from the heat and slowly pour in the eggs in a steady stream, stirring soup constantly in a circular motion so the eggs form fine threads.

Serves 6.

Curried Zucchini Soup

1 tbs safflower oil	3 cups chicken or vegetable broth
2 onions, sliced	
1 garlic clove, minced, optional	herb salt to taste
	dash of cayenne
1 tbs curry powder	¼ tsp grated lemon rind
6 small zucchini, sliced	
	1 cup plain yogurt
1 zucchini, unsliced	2 tbs chopped parsley

Heat oil in a saucepan and sauté onions and garlic over low heat until soft. Stir in curry powder and cook for 2 minutes longer. Stir in sliced zucchini. Add broth, cover, and simmer for 10 minutes, or until zucchini are tender. Stir in herb salt, cayenne, and lemon rind. Puree in batches in blender. Refrigerate until well chilled.

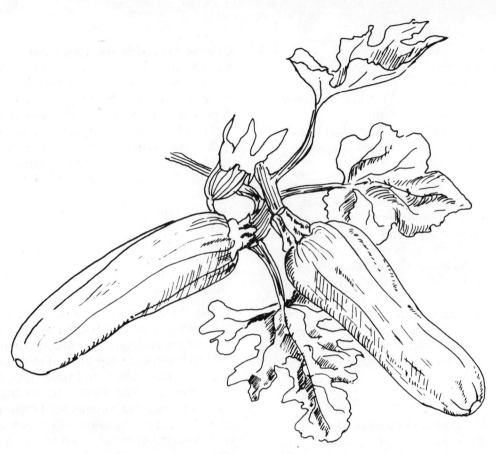

Then cut one zucchini into thin matchstick pieces. Steam in a rack over boiling water for 2 minutes. Chill. Just before serving, stir yogurt into soup and correct seasonings. Ladle into soup bowls and garnish each serving with a spoonful of steamed zucchini and a sprinkling of chopped parsley.

Note: The soup may also be served hot. Reheat before adding yogurt.

Serves 4 to 6.

Fish Potage

1 tbs safflower oil	herb salt and pepper to taste
1 garlic clove, minced	
1 onion, chopped	1 tsp grated lemon rind
2 celery stalks, chopped	dash of Tabasco
2 scallions, cut in ¼-inch pieces	1 tsp tamari
	1 lb halibut, or any firm white fish, skinned, boned, and cut in small pieces
3 cups Italian coarse-chopped plum tomatoes	
½ cup dry white wine *or* vegetable broth	
1 bay leaf	3 tbs chopped parsley

Heat oil in a heavy soup pot. Sauté garlic, onion, celery, and scallions until soft. Add tomatoes, wine, bay leaf, herb salt, pepper, lemon rind, Tabasco, and tamari. Cover and simmer for 20 minutes. Add fish and cook, covered, 12 minutes longer, or until fish is done. Stir in parsley right before serving. For an extra touch, toast 4 slices of whole wheat bread. Place one slice of the toast in each of 4 soup bowls. Ladle soup over toast.

Serves 4.

Gazpacho with Shrimp

1 garlic clove, minced	1 tsp Bronner's Broth
1 small red onion, chopped	½ tsp dry mustard
	¼ tsp dill, optional
1 cucumber, peeled, seeded, and chopped	1 tbs safflower oil
	herb salt and pepper to taste
4 tomatoes, peeled and chopped	2 dashes Tabasco, optional
1 green pepper, seeded and chopped	2 tbs vinegar
	1 cup tomato juice or V8 juice

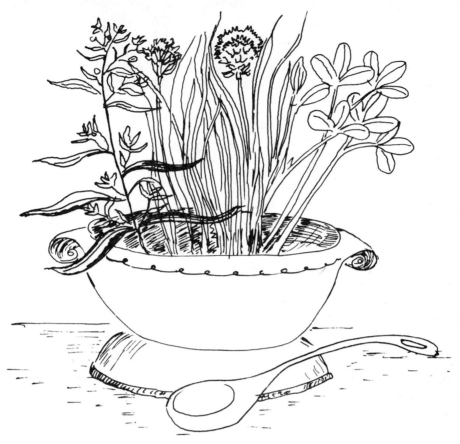

Condiments

½ lb tiny shrimp,
cooked and peeled
1 cucumber, peeled,
seeded, and
chopped

1 onion, chopped
1 green pepper,
chopped

In batches, place all ingredients, except condiments, in blender and purée until smooth. Pour into a bowl and refrigerate until icy cold. Ladle into soup bowls and pass condiments separately.
Serves 4.

Green Herb Gazpacho

3 cucumbers, peeled,
seeded, and
chopped
1 garlic clove
4 scallions, chopped
1 cup watercress
leaves
½ cup parsley sprigs,
stems removed
2 tbs fresh dill or 1 tsp
dried dill

herb salt to taste
pinch of cayenne
dash of Tabasco
3 tbs white wine
vinegar
1 tbs safflower oil
2 cups chicken or
vegetable broth
2 cups yogurt

Condiments

2 tomatoes, chopped
5 scallions, chopped

¼ cup parsley,
chopped

In batches, place all ingredients, except condiments, in blender and blend until smooth. Pour into a bowl and refrigerate until well chilled. Pour into soup bowls and pass condiments separately.
Serves 4 to 6.

Hearty Vegetable Soup

½ cup dried pinto
beans
2 cups water
1 tbs safflower oil
1 garlic clove, minced
1 onion, chopped
2 leeks, sliced
3 cups V8 juice or
tomato juice
4 cups chicken or
vegetable broth
1 cup water
½ cup dry white wine,
optional

4 celery stalks, sliced
¼-inch thick
1 turnip, diced
2 small zucchini,
sliced ¼-inch thick
1 tsp basil
1 tsp marjoram
1 tbs Bronner's Broth
1 cup cabbage,
shredded
¼ cup parsley,
chopped
herb salt and pepper
to taste

½ cup brown rice
4 carrots, sliced
¼-inch thick

½ cup Parmesan
cheese, grated
fresh

Soak beans in water to cover overnight. In the morning, drain them and cook in 2 cups of water for 1½ hours or until barely tender. Drain beans. Heat oil in a large soup pot. Sauté garlic, onion, and leeks over low heat until soft. Add V8 or tomato juice, broth, water, and wine. Bring to a boil. Stir in rice. Reduce heat, cover, and simmer 40 minutes. Add carrots, celery, turnip, zucchini, basil, marjoram, and Bronner's Broth. Simmer 20 minutes. Add cabbage and cook 5 minutes longer, or until cabbage is soft. Stir in parsley and season to taste with herb salt and pepper. Ladle soup into large bowls and sprinkle with Parmesan cheese.

This recipe is only an introduction to the wide world of vegetable soups. Substitute or add any fresh seasonal vegetables making sure to cook each vegetable only until it is tender, not mushy. Experiment with barley or millet instead of rice. Try lentils, kidney beans, or soybeans instead of pinto beans. Cooked chicken, fish, or tofu may be added during the last 5 minutes of cooking.
Serves 8.

Lentil Soup

1 cup dried lentils
2 tbs safflower oil
1 to 2 garlic cloves,
  minced
2 onions, chopped
2 celery stalks,
  chopped
1 qt water
2 cups tomato juice
1 cup white wine
1 tbs Bronner's Broth

1 to 2 tbs tamari to
  taste
1 tsp basil
¼ cup brown rice
2 carrots, sliced
2 cups spinach, stems
  removed and torn
  into bite-size pieces
herb salt and pepper
  to taste
3 tbs chopped parsley

Place lentils in a bowl and cover with water. Let soak 1 hour, then drain. Heat oil in a large soup pot. Sauté garlic, onions, and celery over low heat until soft. Add lentils, water, tomato juice, white wine, Bronner's Broth, tamari, basil, and rice. Bring to a boil. Reduce heat, cover, and simmer for 1 hour. Add carrots and simmer for 20 minutes. Add spinach, herb salt, and pepper. Cook just until spinach is wilted. Stir in parsley.

If making ahead, stir in spinach and parsley when reheating. If soup becomes too dry, add more water or tomato juice.
Serves 6.

Quick Tomato Herb Soup

4 cups tomato juice
  (the thicker, the
  better)
1 tbs Bronner's Broth
2 tbs honey
1 tbs cider vinegar

1 tsp cinnamon (or
  more to taste)
¼ tsp savory, thyme,
  or basil, crushed
  fine

Place all ingredients in a saucepan, cover, and heat just to boiling. Let stand off the heat for 20 minutes. Serve in mugs.

Children enjoy this soup with popcorn floating on top of the soup. May also be topped with a spoonful of yogurt and a sprinkling of chopped chives. Flavor improves if made ahead and refrigerated for 24 hours. Reheat before serving.
Serves 4.

Sorrel Soup

1 tbs. safflower oil
1 onion, chopped
1 pound sorrel,
  chopped
5 cups chicken or
  vegetable broth
2 tbs powdered milk
herb salt to taste

dash of white pepper
½ cup plain yogurt
1 small cucumber,
  peeled, seeded,
  and diced
2 tbs chopped chives
2 hard-boiled eggs,
  chopped

Heat oil in a saucepan and sauté onion very slowly until soft. Add sorrel and mix well. Add broth and bring to a boil. Remove from heat and let stand, covered, for 20 minutes. Stir in powdered milk, herb salt, and white pepper. Purée in batches in blender until very smooth. Pour into a bowl and refrigerate until well chilled. Ladle soup into bowls and garnish each serving with a spoonful of yogurt and a sprinkling of chives, cucumber, and hard-boiled egg.
Serves 6.

Icy Yogurt Salad Soup

3 scallions, minced
6 radishes, chopped
2 cucumbers, peeled,
  seeded, and
  chopped

½ cup fresh dill,
  chopped
1 to 2 garlic cloves,
  minced
herb salt to taste

¼ cup parsley,   pinch of cayenne
  chopped   1 qt plain yogurt

Place all chopped vegetables, herbs, and garlic in a bowl. Mix well with herb salt and cayenne. Let stand for 10 minutes. Stir in yogurt. Cover and refrigerate until icy cold. Thin the soup, if desired, with a little water.
  Serves 4.

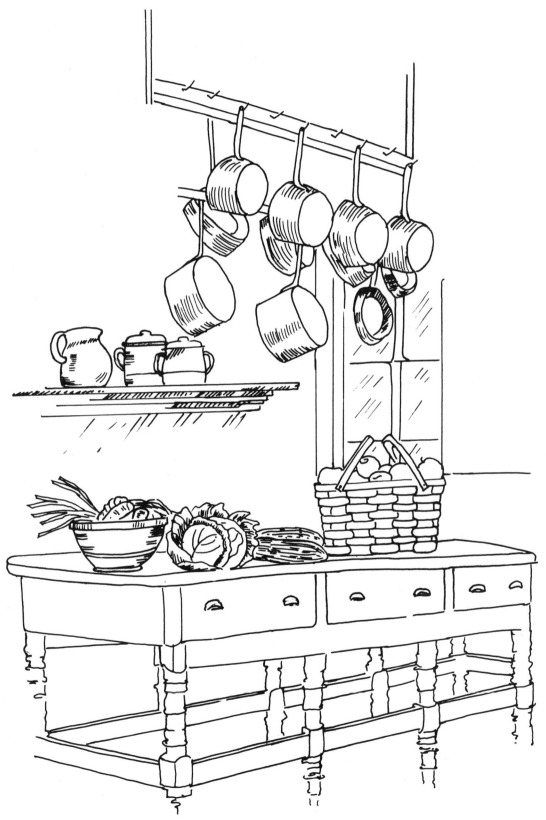

3
The Salad Bowl

The Salad Bar

Boston lettuce
romaine lettuce
red-leaf lettuce
spinach leaves
cabbage, red or green, chopped
  coarse
carrot tops
beet greens
turnip greens
escarole
curly endive
watercress sprigs
parsley sprigs

Choose four or five different greens from the above list—other seasonal favorites may be added if desired. Wash and dry greens, tear into bite-size pieces, and refrigerate until well chilled. Toss greens together in a large salad bowl and place on the table. Offer a choice of two or three dressings and any of the following vegetables, served in separate bowls or arranged decoratively on a large platter.

raw beets, peeled and grated
carrots, grated
celery root, peeled and grated
  (sprinkled with lemon juice)
cucumbers, sliced (peel only if
  waxed)
scallions, minced, *or* red onion rings,
  sliced
Jerusalem artichokes, sliced
zucchini, sliced or grated
mushrooms, sliced
radishes, sliced or cut in roses
green pepper rings
artichoke hearts
tomato wedges or cherry tomatoes
sprouts—alfalfa, mung bean, *or* lentil

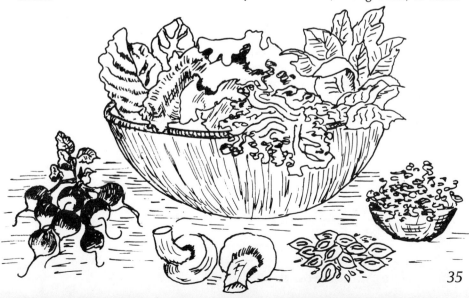

Additional accompaniments may include:

Swiss or Cheddar cheese, grated or cut in julienne strips	chick peas
	sunflower seeds
	fresh dill or basil, chopped
hard-boiled eggs, chopped	croutons

To make croutons: Cut whole wheat bread into small cubes. Place on a cookie sheet and bake in a 275 degree oven for 30 minutes, or until bread is dry and crisp. Turn once while baking. Cool and store in airtight containers. These croutons may not have a typical buttery taste, but no one will notice once they are tossed into the salad.

Celery Root Remoulade

3 medium celery knobs (also known as celeriac)	1½ tbs Dijon mustard
	lemon juice to taste
4 tbs chopped parsley	herb salt and pepper to taste
¼ cup mayonnaise	1 tbs capers, optional
¾ cup plain yogurt	

Peel celery knobs and cut into very thin slices. Then cut slices into thin matchstick pieces. Mix celery root with parsley and place in a bowl. Combine mayonnaise, yogurt, Dijon mustard, lemon juice, herb salt, pepper, and capers. Toss celery root with the dressing, cover, and refrigerate until well chilled. To serve, place salad on a bed of Boston lettuce leaves.

Serves 6.

Chef Salad au Natural

½ head romaine lettuce	2 tomatoes, cut in sixths
1 small head Boston lettuce	3 radishes, sliced thin
1 cup watercress, tough stems removed	1 red onion, sliced
	1 green pepper, cut in rings
1 chicken breast, cooked, skinned, and boned	2 hard-boiled eggs, quartered
6 oz Swiss cheese	1 cup alfalfa sprouts
½ lb artichoke hearts, cooked	salad dressing

Tear lettuce and watercress into bite-size pieces. Place in the bottom of a large salad bowl. Cut chicken and cheese into thin strips. Decoratively arrange chicken, cheese, artichoke hearts, tomatoes, radishes, onion, green pepper, and eggs on top of the lettuce. Sprinkle alfalfa sprouts over the salad. At the table, toss salad with your favorite dressing.

For individual salads, use 4 to 6 large dinner plates and arrange the ingredients on each one as directed above. Pass dressing on the side.

Serves 4 to 6.

Chiffonnade Salad with Pickled Beets

½ cup chicken broth	2 heads Belgian endive
⅓ cup red wine vinegar	1 bunch watercress, tough stems removed
1 stick cinnamon	
8 cloves	
½ tsp herb salt	3 hard-boiled eggs, chopped
1–2 tbs honey	
1 bay leaf	2 tbs chopped parsley
1 bunch beets, cooked and peeled	2 tbs chopped scallions
6 to 8 romaine lettuce leaves	favorite oil and vinegar dressing
6 to 8 Boston lettuce leaves	

Place chicken broth, vinegar, cinnamon stick, cloves, herb salt, honey, and bay leaf in a saucepan and bring to a boil. Cover and simmer for 10 minutes. Strain through a fine sieve. Cut beets into julienne strips. Toss beets with the dressing and let cool. Cover and refrigerate for 24 hours. Drain well. Shred lettuce into thin strips. Tear watercress into bite-size pieces. Cut endive into ½-inch pieces and separate the rings. Place lettuce, watercress, endive, and three-quarters of the eggs in a salad bowl. Toss with your favorite oil and vinegar dressing. Place salad on a large platter and arrange pickled beets in the center. Sprinkle with parsley, scallions, and remaining chopped eggs.

Serves 6.

Chinese Sprout Salad

Salad	*Dressing*
1 small head Boston lettuce	3 tbs cider vinegar
	1 tbs tamari

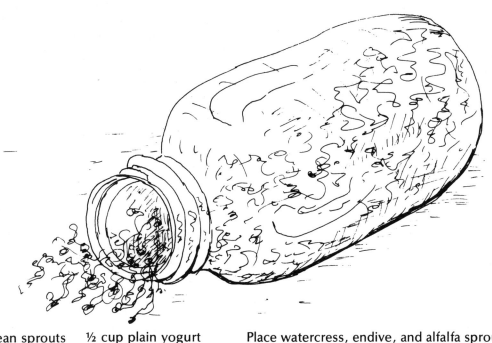

2 cups bean sprouts
½ lb mushrooms, sliced
6 radishes, sliced
½ green pepper, sliced
6 water chestnuts, sliced
4 scallions, minced
1 tbs sesame seeds, optional

½ cup plain yogurt
2 tbs mayonnaise
½ tsp honey
2 tbs chopped chives
1 tbs chopped parsley
pinch of powdered ginger
1 garlic clove, pressed, optional

Mix together all dressing ingredients and refrigerate until well chilled. Tear lettuce into bite-size pieces and mix with the sprouts, mushrooms, radishes, green pepper, water chestnuts, scallions, and sesame seeds. Toss with dressing right before serving.

Serves 6.

Belgian Endive and Watercress Salad

1 bunch watercress, tough stems removed
6 heads Belgian endive

1 cup alfalfa sprouts
vinaigrette dressing

Cut watercress into 1-inch pieces. Cut endive in half lengthwise, discard stem ends, then cut into 1-inch pieces. Wash and dry watercress and endive; refrigerate until crisp and chilled.

Place watercress, endive, and alfalfa sprouts in a salad bowl and toss lightly with vinaigrette dressing right before serving. Serve as a light and elegant salad to complement a hearty main course.

Serves 4 to 6.

Greek Salad

1 head romaine lettuce
2 cucumbers, sliced thin
1 red onion, cut in rings
1 green pepper, cut in rings
8 radishes, sliced thin
1 pint cherry tomatoes, cut in half

4 scallions, minced
6 ounces Feta cheese, crumbled
12 black olives, pitted
2 tbs chopped parsley
½ tsp oregano, crushed
freshly ground pepper
vinaigrette dressing

Tear lettuce into bite-size pieces and arrange in a mound on a large serving platter. Along the inside edge of the lettuce, make a ring of overlapping cucumber slices. Slightly within the cucumbers, make another ring of red onions, peppers and radishes. Mix together the cherry tomatoes, scallions, and feta cheese. Place mixture in the center of the platter. Garnish with olives and sprinkle the entire salad

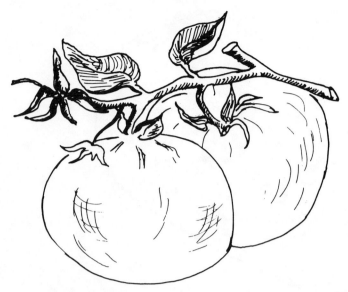

with parsley, oregano, and freshly ground pepper. (It now looks gorgeous!) Cover and refrigerate until well chilled. Pour vinaigrette dressing over the salad at serving time, but do not toss.

Serves 6.

Herbed Cottage Cheese and Cucumber Salad

1 cucumber, peeled, seeded, and diced	4 cups low-fat cottage cheese
2 scallions, minced	½ cup plain yogurt
2 tbs parsley, chopped	½ tsp tarragon or 1 tsp dill
4 radishes, chopped fine	herb salt and pepper to taste
2 tbs chives, chopped	

Mix all ingredients together and refrigerate until well chilled. Serve on a bed of lettuce or inside hollowed-out tomatoes. Garnish with parsley sprigs.

Serves 6.

Marinated Tomatoes

4 tomatoes, sliced	¼ cup safflower oil
1 cucumber, peeled, if waxed, and sliced	2 to 3 tbs honey
1 small red onion, sliced	1 tbs fresh basil, chopped, or 1 tsp dried basil
1 green pepper, cut in rings	2 tbs chopped parsley
½ cup red wine vinegar	1 tbs chopped chives
	herb salt and pepper to taste

Mix tomatoes, cucumbers, onion and green pepper together in a bowl. Combine remaining ingredients and pour over vegetables. Cover and refrigerate for 2 hours. Serve salad on a bed of lettuce.

Serves 4–6.

Mexican Salad

1 garlic clove	1 pimento, cut in thin strips
1 head romaine lettuce, shredded	8 black pitted olives
1 red onion, sliced	2 cups chicken, cooked, skinned, boned, and diced
1 green pepper, cut in thin strips	*or* 2 cups shrimp, cooked and peeled
1 cucumber, peeled, if waxed, and sliced	2 oz Cheddar cheese, grated
3 tomatoes, cut in sixths	2 tbs chopped parsley
2 to 3 mild or hot canned green chili peppers, cut in thin strips	1 avocado, sliced
	oil and vinegar dressing

Rub a large salad bowl with garlic. Place shredded lettuce in the bowl and toss with the red onion, green pepper, cucumber, tomatoes, chili peppers, and pimento. Scatter olives and chicken or shrimp over the top. Garnish with grated cheese, parsley, and avocado. Toss with favorite salad dressing right before serving. Delicious with warm corn tortillas on the side.

To make individual salads, arrange ingredients as directed on 4 large dinner plates. Pass dressing on the side.

Serves 4.

Crunchy Raw Vegetable Salad

A delicious, main-course salad for a warm summer night. Serve with bread and cheese.

1 garlic clove	½ cup broccoli, broken in tiny florets
½ head romaine lettuce	
1 head Boston lettuce	¼ cup parsley, cut in small sprigs
1 cup spinach, stems removed	1 cucumber, sliced
1 cup watercress, cut in 1-inch pieces	1 zucchini, sliced
½ cup cauliflower, broken in tiny	6 scallions, minced
	1 cup alfalfa sprouts
	salad dressing

florets
1 carrot, grated
1 raw beet, peeled
  and grated

4 radishes, grated

Rub a very large salad bowl with garlic. Tear lettuce and spinach into bite-size pieces and place in the bowl. Add the watercress, cauliflower, broccoli, parsley, cucumber, zucchini, scallions, and sprouts. Toss with dressing. Garnish with grated carrots, beets, and radishes.

For additional protein, toss 2 ounces sunflower seeds with the salad. Garnish with 3 hard-boiled eggs, quartered, and/or a mound of cottage cheese in the center of the salad.

Note: Ingredients may be added or omitted at will, according to seasonal specialties and personal preferences. Just remember not to toss the beets or the whole salad will turn red.

Serves 6 to 8.

Salad Niçoise

1 head Boston lettuce
1 12-oz can
  water-packed tuna,
  drained
1 pound green beans,
  cooked
½ pound artichoke
  hearts
3 tomatoes, cut in
  sixths
4 hard-boiled eggs,
  quartered

12 black pitted olives
6 green pepper rings
12 thin red onion
  rings
1 cup alfalfa sprouts
2 tbs. chopped parsley
½ tsp basil
herb salt and pepper
vinaigrette dressing

Make a bed of lettuce leaves on a large platter. Break tuna into chunks and place in the center of the platter. Arrange the beans and artichoke hearts in clumps around the tuna. Garnish platter with tomatoes, eggs, olives, pepper rings, onion rings, and alfalfa sprouts. (Give your artistic talents free rein as you create this edible work of art.) Sprinkle crushed basil, parsley, herb salt and pepper over the salad. Pass vinaigrette dressing on the side.

Serves 6.

Seafood Salad

1½ lb cooked and
  peeled

1 tbs lemon juice
½ tsp dry mustard

shellfish—crab,
  shrimp, and/or
  lobster
1 cup celery, chopped
3 scallions, chopped
2 tbs parsley,
  chopped
⅓ cup plain yogurt
¼ cup ketchup

herb salt and pepper
  to taste
1 head Boston lettuce
1 bunch watercress,
  torn in sprigs
2 cucumbers, sliced
3 tomatoes, sliced
vinaigrette dressing

Mix together the shellfish, celery, scallions, and parsley. In a separate bowl, combine the yogurt, ketchup, lemon juice, dry mustard, herb salt, and pepper. Toss shellfish with the dressing. Cover and refrigerate until well chilled. Tear lettuce into pieces and mound on a platter. Make a ring of watercress around the lettuce. Make an overlapping ring of alternating cucumbers and tomatoes inside the edge of the lettuce. Pile the seafood salad in the center of the ring. Pass vinaigrette dressing on the side.

Serves 6.

Shrimp Salad

1 garlic clove
½ head romaine
  lettuce
½ head Boston lettuce
1 cup spinach, stems
  removed

1 cucumber, sliced
1 cup alfalfa sprouts
10 cherry tomatoes,
  cut in half
3 hard-boiled eggs,
  chopped coarse

½ cup watercress
4 scallions, minced
½ cup celery, chopped
½ green pepper, chopped
1 lb shrimp, cooked and peeled
2 tbs chopped parsley
salad dressing

Rub a large salad bowl with garlic. Tear lettuce, spinach and watercress into bite-size pieces. Place lettuce, spinach, watercress, scallions, celery, green pepper, cucumber, alfalfa sprouts, cherry tomatoes, and eggs in salad bowl. Toss well. Arrange shrimp on top of the salad and sprinkle with parsley. Toss with dressing right before serving.
Serves 4.

Spinach and Sprout Salad

Salad	*Dressing*
10 oz spinach, stems removed	½ cup plain yogurt
2 cups bean sprouts	1 garlic clove, pressed
8 water chestnuts, sliced	1 to 2 tsp Dijon mustard
½ lb mushrooms, sliced	1 tbs lemon juice
3 hard-boiled eggs, chopped	2 tbs safflower oil
4 scallions, minced	herb salt and pepper to taste
	½ tsp honey
	1 tbs chopped chives

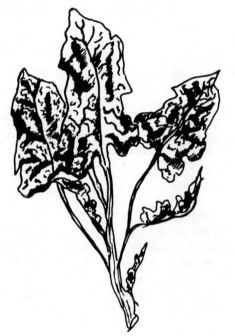

Mix dressing ingredients together and set aside. Tear spinach into bite-size pieces. In a large salad bowl, mix together spinach, sprouts, water chestnuts, mushrooms, eggs, and scallions. Toss salad with dressing and serve at once.
Serves 6.

Tomato-Vegetable Aspic

2 tbs unflavored gelatin	2 tbs lemon juice
4 cups tomato juice	½ cup celery, chopped
⅓ cup onion, chopped	1 tbs scallions, chopped
¼ cup celery leaves, chopped	2 tbs green pepper, chopped
½ tsp herb salt	1 tomato, peeled, seeded, and chopped
1 bay leaf	
2 tsp honey	
1 tbs cider vinegar	1 bunch watercress, in sprigs
4 whole cloves	

Soften gelatin in 1 cup tomato juice. Place 2 cups tomato juice in a saucepan with ⅓ cup onion, ¼ cup celery leaves, herb salt, bay leaf, honey, cider vinegar, and cloves. Bring to a boil and simmer, covered, for 15 minutes. Strain through a fine sieve. Add softened gelatin to hot tomato juice and stir until gelatin is dissolved. Stir in remaining 1 cup tomato juice and lemon juice. Chill until gelatin is thickened, but not set. Stir in chopped celery, scallions, green pepper, and tomato. Pour mixture into a cold wet mold. Refrigerate until set. Unmold onto a platter and decorate outside of the mold with watercress sprigs.

For special occasions, make the aspic in a ring mold and fill the center with Pickled Shrimp (see recipe on p. 000.)
Serves 8.

Salad Dressings

It's not the salads themselves that add unwanted pounds, but rather the high-calorie dressings they are usually drenched in. If salads are tossed well, very little dressing is needed. And don't forget that 2 tablespoons of unsaturated vegetable oil daily are an important part of the Natural Foods Diet.

Your favorite oil-based dressings can be de-calorized by substituting chicken broth, vegetable broth, yogurt, or tomato juice for one-quarter to one-third of the oil called for in the recipe.

Avocado Dressing

1 small avocado, peeled and pitted	3 tbs chopped parsley
1 cup plain yogurt	3 scallions, chopped
2 tbs lemon juice	dash of cayenne
	herb salt to taste

Place all ingredients in blender and blend until very smooth. Serve at once, or cover tightly and refrigerate until needed. If top darkens, stir dressing before serving. Makes 1½ cups.

Bleu Cheese Dressing

1 cup plain yogurt	1 tbs onion
4 ounces bleu cheese	2 tsp tarragon vinegar
1 small garlic clove	herb salt and pepper

Place all ingredients in blender and blend until smooth and creamy. Pour into a bowl, cover, and refrigerate for 24 hours, if possible. The flavor improves on standing. Makes 1½ cups.

Green Herb Dressing

2 egg yolks	4 scallions, chopped
¼ cup tarragon vinegar	2 tbs chives, chopped
1 cup safflower oil	½ tsp dill
½ tsp dry mustard	herb salt and pepper to taste
½ cup parsley, chopped	½ cup plain yogurt
1 cup watercress leaves	

Place egg yolks and vinegar in blender and blend for 5 seconds. With the blender running on "low" speed, slowly pour the oil in a steady stream into the blender. When mixture is thick, add all other ingredients and blend until very smooth. Pour into a jar and refrigerate overnight. Makes 2 cups.

Spicy Oil and Vinegar Dressing

⅔ cup safflower oil	1 tsp Dijon mustard
⅓ cup chicken broth	½ tsp dill
3 to 4 tbs cider vinegar	1 tsp minced parsley
1 tbs red wine vinegar	1 tsp minced chives
1 tbs lemon juice	herb salt and pepper to taste

Place all ingredients in a jar and shake vigorously until well blended. Makes 1⅓ cups.

Tamari Dressing

¾ cup yogurt	1½ tbs tamari, or to taste
3 tbs mayonnaise	

Mix all ingredients together and toss with salad.

Note: Because of the high salt content of this dressing, it should not be used by anyone who has a water-retention problem. Makes 1 cup.

Vinaigrette Dressing

3 tbs vinegar
2 tsp lemon juice
⅓ cup safflower oil
2 tbs chicken broth
1 tsp Dijon mustard,
 optional

herb salt and pepper
 to taste
1 garlic clove,
 pressed, optional

Place all ingredients in a jar and shake until well blended. Makes ⅔ cup.

Yogurt Dressing

1 cup plain yogurt
2 tbs lemon juice *or*
 tarragon vinegar
½ tsp dry mustard
2 tbs chopped parsley
2 tbs chopped chives

1 garlic clove,
 pressed, optional
½ tsp dill
herb salt and pepper
 to taste

Gently stir all ingredients together. Cover

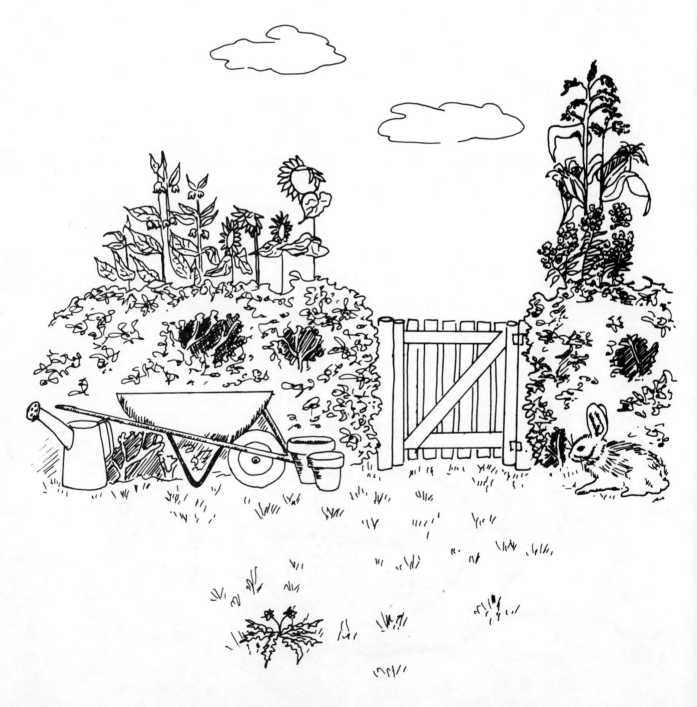

4
From Garden to Table

Fresh vegetables contain a powerhouse of vitamins and minerals, but many of these valuable nutrients are lost by improper handling and cooking methods. Soaking leafy greens or boiling vegetables can wash the C and B vitamins, which are water soluble, right down the drain. With a little bit of care and attention, you can avoid this unnecessary waste and preserve the natural goodness of vegetables.

After picking or purchasing vegetables, wash them quickly, without soaking, dry them, and store in plastic bags in the refrigerator. Cut them into desired shapes and sizes right before cooking so the vitamins will not be destroyed by contact with oxygen.

Steaming and stir-frying are two of the preferred methods for cooking vegetables. To steam, place vegetables in a stainless steel steamer basket in a pot with one inch of boiling water. Cover with a tight-fitting lid and cook over heat that is just hot enough to keep the water bubbling. The liquid that remains in the pot after cooking can be added to a soup or broth.

Stir-frying may be done in a wok, skillet, or heavy pot. Heat a small bit of oil over medium-high heat, then add the vegetables, and stir constantly while cooking.

With both methods, be sure not to overcook the vegetables. Nothing is more unpalatable than vegetables that have been cooked to an unidentifiable mush. No precise timetable can be given for cooking them because so many variables are involved: the age and condition of the vegetables, the size of the pieces, the amount of heat, and the type of pot used. Learn to use the "bite test." Vegetables are done when they are tender-crisp—slightly soft, yet still crunchy.

Vegetables are too delicious and nutritious to be relegated to a place of minor importance. Feature them as the star attraction of a wonderful low-calorie vegetarian meal.

Italian Artichokes

4 artichokes
2 tbs safflower oil
1 garlic clove, minced
1 small onion,
   chopped
1 tbs lemon juice
2 tsp tarragon
   vinegar

1 tbs chopped
   parsley
½ cup chicken
   or vegetable broth
½ cup white wine
½ tsp tarragon
herb salt and pepper
   to taste

Trim stalk from base of artichokes, cut off prickly tops, and remove tough outer leaves.

Place artichokes on a rack and steam over 1 inch of boiling water for 25 minutes. Cut artichokes into quarters lengthwise and remove inner choke. Heat oil in a saucepan. Sauté garlic and onion until soft. Add remaining ingredients to pan, then stir in artichokes. Cover and simmer for 20 minutes, or until artichokes are tender. To serve, pour juices from pan over artichokes.
Serves 4.

Acorn Squash Souffle

4 small acorn squash
2 tbs butter
3 tbs whole wheat
   pastry flour
1 small onion, cut in
   pieces
½ cup milk
½ cup chicken or
   vegetable broth

¼ tsp ginger
½ tsp cinnamon
sea salt to taste
pinch of cayenne
4 eggs, separated
2 tbs Parmesan
   cheese, grated

Wash squash; turn each on its flat side and cut off the tops horizontally. Remove seeds and fibers. Place squash and tops, cut side down, in a pan containing ½ inch of water. Bake in a 350 degree oven for 1 hour. Remove from oven and cool. Scoop out pulp, reserving shells and discarding tops. Place butter, flour onion, milk, broth, ginger, cinnamon, salt, cayenne, and squash pulp in blender. Blend until smooth. Pour the squash mixture into a saucepan and cook over medium heat, stirring until sauce thickens. Turn mixture into a large bowl and beat in egg yolks, one at a time. Beat egg whites until stiff, but not dry. Fold whites into squash mixture. Place squash shells in a shallow baking dish. Spoon souffle mixture into shells, filling them three-quarters full. Sprinkle with Parmesan cheese. Any extra souffle mixture may be baked in a separate dish. Bake in a preheated 375 degree oven for 25 to 30 minutes, until puffy. Serve at once.
Serves 4.

Stir-Fried Ginger Broccoli

1 bunch broccoli
1 tbs safflower oil
1 garlic clove, minced
1 tsp fresh ginger,
   minced

4 tbs water or chicken
   broth
1 tbs soy sauce

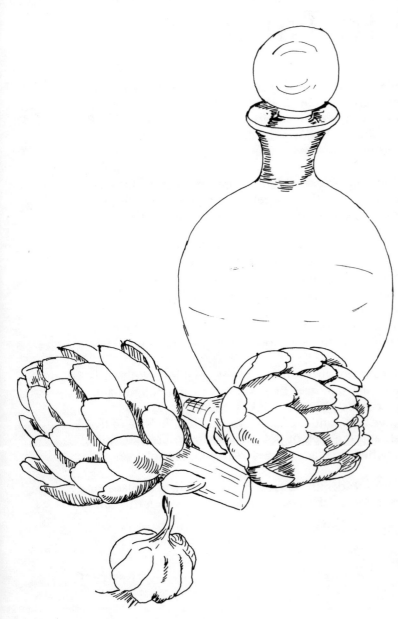

Cut off broccoli florets and slice stems on the diagonal into ¼-inch pieces. Heat oil in a wok or large skillet. Add garlic and ginger and stir-fry for 20 seconds. Add broccoli and cook, stirring, for 2 to 3 minutes. Add water or broth and soy sauce. Cover and steam for 5 to 7 minutes, until broccoli is barely tender.

Variation: For a nice Christmasy touch, add ¼ cup thin-slivered red peppers 2 minutes before broccoli is done.

Serves 4.

Butternut Squash with Honey Apples

2 butternut squash	2 tbs honey
1 tbs butter	1 tbs sherry
1 onion, chopped	1 to 2 tsp cinnamon,
4 tart apples, peeled, cored, and diced	optional
2 tbs apple cider or water	

Cut squash in half and remove seeds and fibers. Place in a baking dish, cut side down, and fill pan with ½ inch of hot water. Bake in a 400 degree oven for 35 minutes. Remove from oven. If necessary, cut bottoms off squash to make a flat edge. Melt butter in a large skillet. Sauté onion over low heat until soft. Add apples and apple cider or water. Cook for 4 minutes. Stir in honey, sherry, and cinnamon. Place squash in a shallow baking dish and fill cavities with apple mixture. Cover bottom of dish with a little water. Return to 400 degree oven for 20 minutes, or until squash is tender.

Serves 4.

Cabbage Stew

2 tbs. safflower oil	1 cup chicken or
2 onions, chopped	vegetable broth
1 garlic clove, minced, optional	1 tbs cider vinegar
2 leeks, sliced	1 tsp thyme
3 carrots, sliced	4 whole cloves
2 potatoes, sliced	herb salt and pepper
1 small head cabbage, cut in wedges, core removed	to taste

Heat oil in a large pot or Dutch oven. Sauté onion, garlic, and leeks until soft. Stir in carrots and potatoes. Place cabbage wedges over sautéed vegetables. Add broth, vinegar, thyme, cloves, herb salt, and pepper. Cover tightly and simmer over low heat for 30 minutes, or until cabbage is tender. Stir occasionally while cooking.

Serves 4.

Stir-Fried Celery and Mushrooms

1 bunch celery	½ lb fresh
2 tbs safflower oil	mushrooms, sliced
1 large onion, chopped	thick
	2 tbs soy sauce

Remove strings from celery stalks and cut into ¾-inch diagonal pieces. Heat oil in a wok or large skillet. Sauté onion for 1 minute. Add celery and mushrooms and stir-fry for 3 to 4 minutes, until celery is tender-crisp. Stir in soy sauce and serve at once.

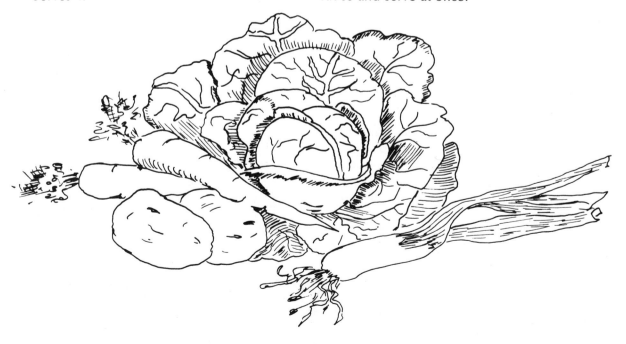

Variation: 2 tbs chopped parsley and 3 tbs toasted slivered almonds may be added at the same time as the soy sauce.

To serve as a main course, stir in 1 lb crab meat or 1 lb raw, peeled shrimp. Cook just until crab is heated through, or shrimp are cooked.

Serves 4.

Chinese Peas and Bean Sprouts

1 lb Chinese snow peas
2 tbs safflower oil
1 onion, chopped
½ lb bean sprouts
8 water chestnuts, sliced
⅔ cup chicken or vegetable broth
2 tbs soy sauce
1 tsp arrowroot or cornstarch

Remove tips and strings from snow peas. If pods are large, cut in half. Heat oil in a wok or large skillet. Sauté onion until soft. Add snow peas and stir-fry for 3 minutes. Add bean sprouts, water chestnuts, and broth. Cover and simmer for 3 to 4 minutes, until peas are barely tender. (They should still go "crunch" when you bite into them.) Mix together the soy sauce and arrowroot or cornstarch to form a paste. Pour over vegetables and cook just until sauce thickens.

Serves 4 to 6.

Creole Summer Squash

2 tbs safflower oil
1 onion, chopped
½ green pepper, chopped
1 garlic clove, minced, optional
2 tomatoes, peeled and chopped coarse
3 zucchini, sliced ¼ inch thick
2 yellow squash, sliced ¼-inch thick
herb salt and pepper to taste

Heat oil in a large skillet. Sauté onion, green pepper, and garlic until soft. Add tomatoes, zucchini, and yellow squash. Simmer over low heat until squash is tender. Stir occasionally. Season to taste with herb salt and pepper.

Serves 4 to 6.

Baked Tomatoes Parmigiana

2 large tomatoes, cut in half
3 tbs fine whole wheat bread crumbs
2 tbs grated Parmesan cheese
1 tbs sesame seeds
2 tbs melted butter
herb salt and pepper to taste

Place tomatoes close together in a shallow baking dish. Mix remaining ingredients together and spread over tops of tomatoes. Cover bottom of pan with some water. Bake in a preheated 375 degree oven for 15 minutes. If necessary, place under broiler to brown tops before serving.

Serves 4.

Ratatouille Crêpes

2 tbs safflower oil
1 garlic clove, minced
1 large onion, sliced
1 green pepper, seeded and cut in thin 1-inch strips
1 eggplant, cut in cubes
2 zucchini, sliced ¼-inch thick
4 tomatoes, peeled and cubed
½ tsp basil
¼ tsp thyme
herb salt and pepper to taste
2 tbs chopped parsley
8 cooked crêpes
4 tbs Parmesan cheese, grated

Heat oil in a large skillet. Sauté garlic and onion until soft. Add green peppers, eggplant, zucchini, tomatoes, basil, thyme, herb salt, and pepper. Stir mixture together, cover, and simmer for 10 minutes. Remove cover and simmer

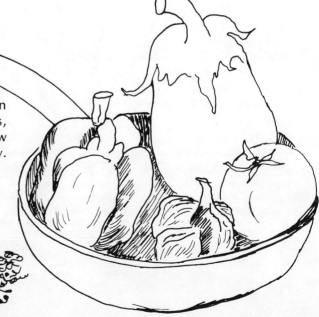

until vegetables are tender and liquid has evaporated. Stir in parsley.

(To make crêpes, follow recipe for Apricot-Orange Crêpes Flambé, (see p.   ), omitting honey and vanilla.)

Place 3 to 4 tablespoons ratatouille in the center of each crêpe. Roll loosely and place in a single layer in a shallow baking dish. Sprinkle with Parmesan cheese. Bake in a preheated 350 degree oven for 20 minutes, or until filling is hot. Place under broiler to brown slightly before serving.

Note: Cold ratatouille makes a delicious snack or hors d'oeuvre when served on toasted pita bread.

Serves 4.

Vegetable Chow Mein

1 cup cauliflower florets
2 tbs safflower oil
6 scallions, cut in 1-inch pieces
3 celery stalks, cut in ¼-inch pieces
3 carrots, sliced thin
1 green pepper, seeded, cut in thin strips
2 cups cabbage, shredded
½ cup bamboo shoots, sliced thin
1 tbs sherry
2 tbs soy sauce
1 tsp honey
herb salt and pepper to taste
¾ cup chicken or vegetable broth
2 tsp arrowroot or cornstarch
2 tbs water

Steam cauliflower for 6 to 7 minutes, or until barely tender. Heat oil in a wok or large skillet. Add scallions, celery, carrots, and green pepper. Stir-fry for 5 minutes. Add cabbage, bamboo shoots, cauliflower, sherry, soy sauce, honey, herb salt, pepper, and broth. Cover and simmer 5 minutes. Mix together arrowroot or cornstarch and water to form a paste. Stir into vegetables and cook just until sauce is thickened. Serve vegetables on a bed of brown rice.

Note: Other vegetables in season may be substituted for the ones given.

Serves 4.

Brown Rice and Vegetable Pilaf

2 tbs safflower oil
1 garlic clove, minced
1 onion, chopped
1 cup brown rice
¼ cup white wine
dash of Tabasco
herb salt and pepper to taste
2 cups vegetable or chicken broth
2 tsp tamari
pinch of saffron or tumeric
1 cup artichoke hearts, cut in small pieces (frozen may be used)
1 cup mushrooms, sliced
½ cup green peas cooked (may use frozen, defrosted ones)
2 tbs chopped parsley

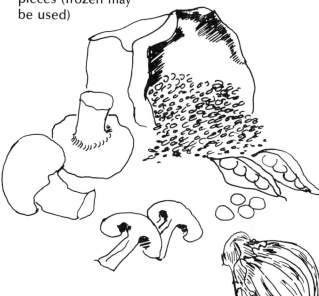

Heat oil in a saucepan. Add garlic and onion and sauté until onion is soft. Add rice and cook, stirring, for 1 minute. Add broth, tamari and saffron or tumeric. Boil for 2 minutes. Reduce heat, cover, and simmer for 40 minutes. Add artichoke hearts, white wine, Tabasco sauce, herb salt, pepper, and mushrooms. Cover and simmer for 10 minutes longer. Stir in peas and parsley. Let stand off the heat a few minutes before serving.

Serves 4.

Vegetarian Bleu Cheese Delight

4 small zucchini
2 tbs safflower oil
1 garlic clove, minced
1 onion, chopped
½ lb mushrooms, quartered
4 cups romaine lettuce, shredded
1 carrot, grated
1 raw beet, peeled and grated
2 tomatoes, cut in sixths
1 cup Bleu Cheese Dressing (see Index)

2 cups hot, cooked
  brown rice
1 green pepper,
  seeded and cut in
  thin strips

1 cup alfalfa sprouts

Quarter zucchini lengthwise, then cut into ½-inch pieces. Heat oil in a skillet. Sauté garlic and onion until soft. Add zucchini and mushrooms and cook until vegetables are tender-crisp. While vegetables are cooking, make a bed of lettuce on four dinner plates. Spoon ½ cup hot rice onto center of the lettuce. Top with hot zucchini mixture. Garnish with green pepper, carrots, beets, and tomatoes. Spoon Bleu Cheese Dressing (see p.   ) over all and top with a sprinkling of alfalfa sprouts. Serve at once.

Serves 4.

Spinach and Wheat Pilaf Casserole

1 box wheat pilaf
  (available at
  supermarkets and
  health food stores)
2 tbs butter
2 onions, chopped
10 oz fresh spinach,
  stems removed,
  torn into small
  pieces
½ tsp thyme

1 tsp basil
2 tbs chopped parsley
herb salt and pepper
  to taste
1 tbs tamari
2 eggs, lightly beaten
4 tbs Parmesan
  cheese, grated
4 oz Monterey Jack or
  Cheddar cheese,
  grated

Prepare wheat pilaf according to directions on package. Place cooked pilaf in the bottom of a casserole dish. Melt butter in a large skillet. Sauté onion until soft. Add spinach and cook just until leaves are wilted. Stir in thyme, basil, parsley, herb salt, pepper, and tamari. Mix in eggs and Parmesan cheese. Place mixture over pilaf in dish. Top with grated cheese. Bake in a 375 degree oven for 30 minutes, or until hot and bubbly.

Serves 4.

5
Main Attractions

Chicken With Artichoke Hearts

1 3½-lb chicken, cut into serving pieces, excess fat removed
2 tbs shallots or scallions, chopped fine
2 tbs whole wheat pastry flour
1 cup chicken broth
¾ cup white wine
12 small white onions, peeled
½ tsp tarragon or rosemary

sea salt and pepper to taste
½ lb frozen artichoke hearts, defrosted
½ lb fresh mushrooms, stems removed
¼ cup chopped parsley

Place chicken, skin side down, in a heavy iron skillet or nonstick pan and cook slowly over medium-low heat until brown on all sides. Remove chicken from pan. Add shallots or scallions and sauté 1 minute. Stir in flour. Slowly add broth and wine, stirring constantly to remove any lumps. Return chicken to skillet and add onions, tarragon or rosemary, sea salt, and pepper. Cover skillet and simmer for 30 minutes. Add artichoke hearts and mushrooms. Cover and continue cooking 15 minutes longer. Stir in parsley right before serving.
Serves 4.

Chicken Kebobs

2 whole chicken breasts, skinned, boned, cut in cubes

Marinade

½ cup soy sauce
2 tbs sherry
2 tbs honey
4 tbs tomato juice
1 garlic clove, minced
1 to 2 tsp fresh ginger, minced
2 scallions, minced
2 green peppers, seeded and cut in 1½-inch squares

½ lb mushrooms, stems removed
12 small white onions, steamed for 3 minutes, then peeled

Mix together marinade ingredients. Pour sauce over cubed chicken and refrigerate for 4 to 6 hours. Thread chicken on skewers alternately with peppers, mushrooms, and onions. Grill over charcoal or broil in the oven, turning once and basting often with reserved marinade.
Serves 4.

Chicken Marengo

1 3½-lb frying chicken, cut into serving pieces, excess fat removed
3 onions, sliced
1 tbs whole wheat pastry flour
1 cup dry white wine

¾ cup chicken broth
2 tbs tomato paste
¼ tsp thyme
½ lb mushrooms, cut in thick slices
2 tbs chopped parsley
sea salt and pepper to taste

Place chicken, skin side down, in a heavy iron skillet or nonstick pan and cook slowly over medium-low heat until brown on all sides. Remove chicken from pan and add onions. Sauté for 3 minutes. Sprinkle with flour. Stir well and slowly add wine, chicken broth, tomato paste, and thyme, stirring until lumps are gone. Bring mixture to a boil. Add reserved chicken and mix with sauce. Cover and simmer for 30 minutes. Add mushrooms and parsley. Continue cooking for 15 minutes. Season to taste with sea salt and pepper.
Serves 4.

Chinese Chicken and Snow Peas

2 tbs safflower oil
1 garlic clove, minced
1 tsp fresh ginger, minced
2 chicken breasts, skinned, boned, cut in 1-inch cubes
4 scallions, cut in 1-inch pieces
¼ cup bamboo shoots, cut in thin strips

¼ cup water chestnuts, sliced
½ lb snow peas, cut in half if large
2 tbs soy sauce
2 tbs sherry
½ cup chicken broth
2 tsp arrowroot or cornstarch
2 tbs water

Heat oil in a wok or large skillet. Add garlic and ginger and stir-fry for 15 seconds. Add chicken and stir-fry for 2 minutes, or until chicken turns white. Remove chicken from pan with a slotted spoon. Add scallions, bamboo shoots, water chestnuts, and snow peas to wok. Stir-fry for 3 to 4 minutes. Add soy sauce, sherry, chicken broth, and reserved chicken. Mix arrowroot or cornstarch with water to form a paste. Stir into chicken and cook, stirring, just until sauce is thickened. Serve at once with brown rice.
Serves 4.

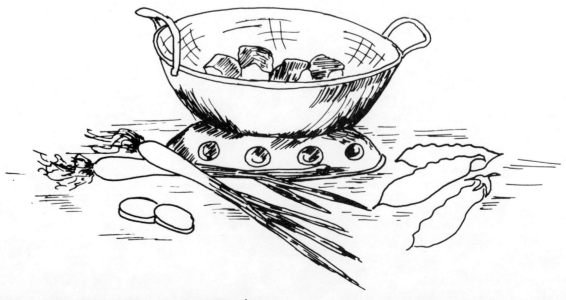

Cold, Spicy Lemon Chicken

6 dried Chinese black mushrooms
3 small chicken breasts, skinned and boned
1 tbs soy sauce
2 green peppers
1 hot green pepper (use a small one if very hot)
2 tbs safflower oil
1 tsp fresh ginger, minced
2 tsp arrowroot or cornstarch
4 tbs lemon juice
4 tbs chicken broth
1 tbs grated lemon rind
1 to 2 dashes of Tabasco
1 head romaine lettuce, shredded

Soak mushrooms in warm water to cover for 30 minutes. Drain and squeeze dry. Remove hard stems and slice mushrooms into thin strips. Cut chicken into thin strips, about 2 inches long. Mix chicken with soy sauce and set aside. Discard seeds and membranes from pepper and cut into very thin strips, 2-inches long. Heat oil until quite hot in a wok or large skillet. Add ginger and stir-fry for 5 seconds. Add chicken, mushrooms, and peppers. Stir-fry just until chicken turns white, about 2 minutes. Mix arrowroot or cornstarch with lemon juice and chicken broth. Add to wok and cook, stirring, until sauce is thickened. Stir in lemon rind and Tabasco. Pour into a bowl and let cool to room temperature. Serve on a bed of chilled, shredded romaine lettuce. May also be served hot with brown rice.

Serves 4.

Tarragon Chicken

1 3½-lb chicken, quartered, excess fat removed

Marinade

2 tbs safflower oil
¼ cup lemon juice
1 tbs chopped chives
1 tsp tarragon
1 tbs chopped parsley
herb salt and pepper to taste

Place chicken in a bowl. Mix all other ingredients together. Rub sauce on chicken and let marinate in the refrigerator for several hours or overnight. Place chicken on a roasting rack in a shallow pan. Pour marinade over chicken. Bake in a pre-heated 350 degree oven for 1 hour, basting often with juices in the pan.

Serves 4.

Chinese Ginger Bass

4 dried Chinese black mushrooms
1 cup cooked brown rice
4 scallions, minced
1½ tsp fresh ginger, minced
3 tbs soy sauce
1 3-lb sea bass, cleaned, head and tail left on
1½ tbs cider vinegar
½ tsp honey
1 tbs safflower oil
¼ tsp pepper

Soak mushrooms in water to cover for 30 minutes. Drain and squeeze dry; slice thinly, discarding hard stems. Combine mushrooms, rice, half the minced scallions, half the ginger and 1 tbs soy sauce. Stuff bass with mixture. With a sharp knife, score bass lightly on both sides making diagonal cuts through the skin. Place fish on an ovenproof plate. Mix together the remaining scallions, ginger, vinegar, honey, oil, and pepper. Pour mixture over fish. Place plate on a rack in a large kettle or steamer, with 1 to 2 inches of boiling water on the bottom. Cover and steam for 20 minutes, or until fish flakes easily when tested with a fork.

Serves 4–6.

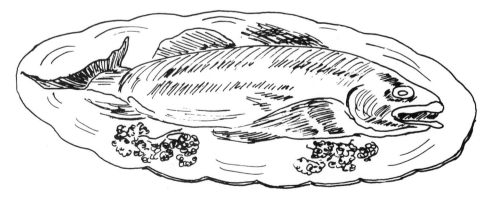

Fillet of Sole Bonne Femme

1½ lb sole fillets
sea salt and pepper to taste
1 tsp dill
2 tbs chopped parsley
2 tbs chopped chives
¼ cup dry white wine
2 tbs lemon juice
12 oz mushrooms, sliced thick
1 tbs butter
paprika

Rub fish on both sides with sea salt, pepper, and dill. Place in a single layer in a shallow baking dish. Sprinkle with parsley, chives, white wine, and lemon juice. Place mushrooms on top and around fish. Dot with butter and sprinkle with paprika. Bake in a preheated 350 degree oven for 15 to 20 minutes, basting often with juices in the pan. Transfer fish to a heated serving platter and pour juices from pan over fish. Garnish platter with parsley sprigs and lemon wedges.

Serves 4.

Grilled Halibut

1½ lb halibut steaks

Marinade

1 tbs safflower oil
2 tbs lemon juice
½ cup dry white wine
2 tbs soy sauce
2 scallions, minced
2 tbs parsley, minced
¼ tsp tarragon
sea salt and pepper to taste

Place fish in a shallow dish. Mix marinade ingredients together and pour over fish. Turn to coat both sides with the marinade. Refrigerate for at least 2 hours. Grill fish over charcoal for 20 minutes, turning once, or broil for 15 to 20 minutes. Baste with remaining marinade while cooking. Place fish on a warm platter and garnish with parsley springs and lemon wedges.

Serves 4.

Baked Salmon with Cucumber-Dill Sauce

1 2-lb salmon steak
2 tbs lemon juice
2 tbs white wine
paprika
1 lemon, cut in wedges
1 bunch watercress, cut in sprigs

Cucumber-Dill Sauce

1 small cucumber, peeled and seeded
2 tsp lemon juice
1 tbs fresh dill or 1 tsp
¾ cup plain yogurt
2 tbs mayonnaise
2 tbs chopped parsley
2 tbs chopped chives
dried
herb salt to taste
pinch of cayenne

Rub salmon all over with lemon juice and wine. Place in a shallow baking dish and sprinkle with paprika. Bake in a preheated 350 degree oven for 20 minutes. Place under broiler to brown lightly. Place on a serving platter, garnished with watercress and lemon wedges. Pass Cucumber-Dill Sauce in a separate bowl. While fish is cooking, grate cucumber and squeeze dry. (In fact, rub the excess cucumber liquid on your face for a quick, soothing, and natural facial.) Mix cucumber with all remaining ingredients. Refrigerate sauce until serving time.

Serves 4–6.

Shrimp Italian

2 tbs safflower oil
1 garlic clove, minced
½ cup onion, chopped
½ cup celery, chopped
½ lb mushrooms, sliced
2 tbs tomato paste
½ tsp rosemary, crushed
½ tsp basil, crushed
1 bay leaf
2 dashes of Tabasco
herb salt and pepper to taste

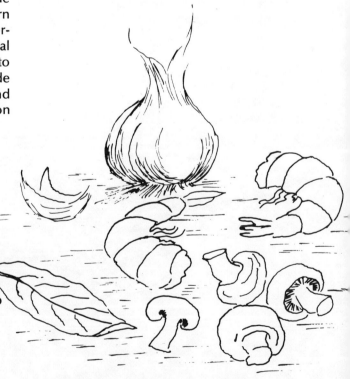

1 1-pound 3-oz can
Italian plum
tomatoes drained,
chopped coarse

1½ lb raw shrimp,
shelled
1 green pepper, cut in
1-inch cubes

Heat oil in a saucepan. Sauté garlic, onion, and celery for 5 minutes. Add mushrooms and cook 1 minute longer. Add tomatoes, tomato paste, rosemary, basil, bay leaf, Tabasco, herb salt, and pepper. Simmer, uncovered, for 20 minutes. Add shrimp and green pepper. Simmer for 10 minutes. Serve over brown rice along with a big green salad.

Sole Surprise

8 small sole fillets
1 onion, sliced thin
2 tomatoes, peeled
and sliced
8 mushrooms, sliced
2 tbs parsley,
chopped

½ tsp dill
herb salt and pepper
to taste
2 tsp butter
4 tsp dry white wine
cooking parchment
paper

Cut parchment paper into 4 8-by-14-inch rectangles. Place 2 sole fillets in the middle of each paper. Cover fish with a layer of onions, tomatoes, and mushrooms. Sprinkle with parsley, dill, herb salt, and pepper. Dot each with ½ tsp butter. Sprinkle each with 1 tsp wine. Fold parchment paper together, tucking ends under, to make tight little packages. Place on a shallow dish. Bake in a preheated 350 degree oven for 25 minutes. To serve, place one package on each plate and slit open the tops to let steam escape.

Serves 4.

Stuffed Lobsters

1 tbs safflower oil
1 large onion,
chopped
2 celery stalks,
chopped
1½ cups cucumber,
peeled, seeded,
and diced in small
cubes
¼ tsp thyme
¼ tsp tarragon
2 slices whole wheat
bread, cut in small
cubes

2 tbs chopped parsley
1 egg, lightly beaten
sea salt and pepper to
taste
4 lobsters (1¼ lb
each), split and
cleaned
safflower oil
2 lemons, cut in half
parsley sprigs

Heat oil in a skillet. Sauté onion and celery until soft. Stir in cucumber, thyme, tarragon, bread cubes, and chopped parsley. Remove from heat and add beaten egg, salt, and pepper. Fill the cavity of each lobster with an equal portion of the mixture. Brush tails with oil. Place lobsters on a baking sheet. Bake in a preheated 425 degree oven for 25 minutes. Serve with lemon wedges and parsley sprigs.

Note: Plain steamed or boiled lobsters are a marvelous treat for dieters. They are high in protein and low in calories. Serve with lemon wedges and forego the melted butter.

Serves 4.

Quick Cheese Souffle

3 tbs butter
4 tbs whole wheat
pastry flour
½ tsp sea salt
pinch of cayenne
½ tsp dry mustard
1 cup milk, scalded

4 oz sharp Cheddar
cheese, cut in small
cubes
4 egg yolks
6 egg whites
pinch of cream of
tartar

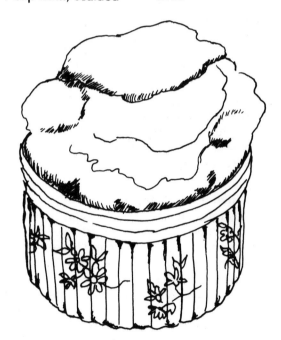

Place butter, flour, sea salt, cayenne, mustard, milk, and cheese in blender. Blend on high speed for 30 seconds, or until well blended. Pour mixture into a saucepan and cook over medium heat, stirring, until sauce thickens. Remove from heat and beat in egg yolks, one at a time. Pour mixture into a large bowl and cool slightly. In separate bowl beat egg whites with cream of tartar until stiff but not dry. Gently fold whites into cheese mixture. Turn into a buttered 1½-qt souffle dish. Bake in a preheated 375 degree oven for 25 to 30 minutes or until puffed and golden. Serve immediately.

Serves 3 to 4.

Pita Pizzas

3 whole pita breads
1½ cups thick tomato sauce or spaghetti sauce
8 oz sharp Cheddar cheese, grated
2 cups mushrooms, sliced
1 cup onion, chopped fine

1 cup green pepper, chopped fine
1 tsp basil, crushed
1 tsp oregano, crushed
herb salt and pepper to taste
4 tbs Parmesan cheese, grated

Slice pita bread around edges and split the halves apart. Place on a cookie sheet. Bake in a preheated 450 degree oven for 2 minutes, or until slightly crispy. Spread tomato sauce over pita bread. Sprinkle with cheese, then mushrooms, onion, green pepper, basil, oregano, herb salt, pepper, and Parmesan cheese. Lower oven to 350 degrees and bake 15 to 20 minutes. Serve with a big green salad, for a quick and easy Sunday night supper. Nondieters will probably want two halves.

Serves 6.

Stir-Fried Broccoli and Tofu

4 pads tofu, cut in small cubes
2 tbs tamari
1 bunch broccoli, cut in bite-size pieces
2 tbs safflower oil
1 garlic clove, minced
1 tsp fresh ginger, minced
½ lb mushrooms, quartered

6 to 8 water chestnuts, sliced
½ cup chicken or vegetable broth
2 tbs sherry
dash of Tabasco
2 tsp cornstarch or arrowroot
2 tbs water
¼ cup slivered toasted almonds

Mix tofu with tamari and marinate for 3 to 4 hours. Steam broccoli for 5 minutes. Heat oil in a wok or large skillet. Add garlic and ginger and stir-fry for 15 seconds. Add broccoli and mushrooms. Cook for 3 minutes, stirring. Add tofu and water chestnuts and mix well with broccoli—stir gently so tofu does not break. Add broth, sherry, and Tabasco. Mix cornstarch or arrowroot and water to form a paste. Stir into wok and cook until sauce thickens. Sprinkle with almonds right before serving.

Serves 4.

Tofu Provençale

2 tbs safflower oil
1 garlic, minced
1 onion, chopped coarse
1 green pepper, chopped coarse
1 eggplant, peeled and diced
3 tomatoes, peeled, coarse chopped

½ lb mushrooms, sliced
1 tsp basil
herb salt and pepper to taste
2 tbs chopped parsley
3 pads tofu, cut in ½-inch cubes

Heat oil in a skillet. Add garlic, onion and green pepper. Sauté for 5 minutes. Add eggplant and cook, stirring, until eggplant is barely tender. Add tomatoes, mushrooms, basil, herb salt, and pepper. Simmer uncovered, for 10 to 15 minutes. Gently stir in parsley and tofu. Cook just until tofu is heated through.

Serves 4.

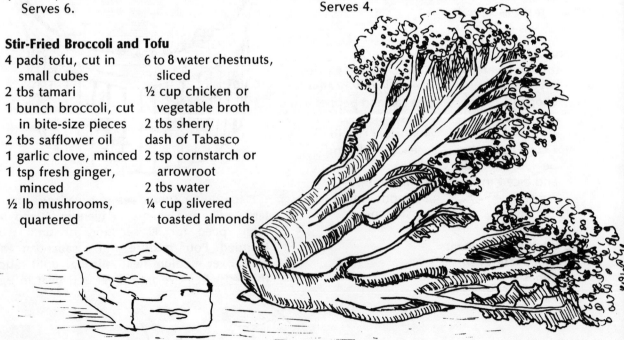

Curried Soybeans

2 tbs safflower oil
1 large onion, chopped
1 green pepper, chopped
1 celery stalk, chopped
2 small apples, cored, peeled, and chopped
1 to 2 tbs curry powder to taste
1 tbs whole wheat pastry flour
1 bay leaf
1 tsp lemon rind
1 tbs lemon juice
2 cups vegetable broth
herb salt to taste
4 cups cooked soybeans
brown rice, cooked

Condiments

chopped green pepper
chopped scallions
chopped cucumber
chopped tomato
chopped hard-boiled eggs
raisins
sunflower seeds or chopped peanuts

Heat safflower oil in a large saucepan. Sauté onion, green pepper, celery, and apples until soft. Stir in curry powder and flour. Cook over low heat for 1 to 2 minutes. Add bay leaf, lemon rind, lemon juice, broth, herb salt, and soybeans. Mix well, cover, and simmer for 20 minutes, stirring occasionally. Serve the curry over brown rice and pass condiments in individual bowls.

Serves 4.

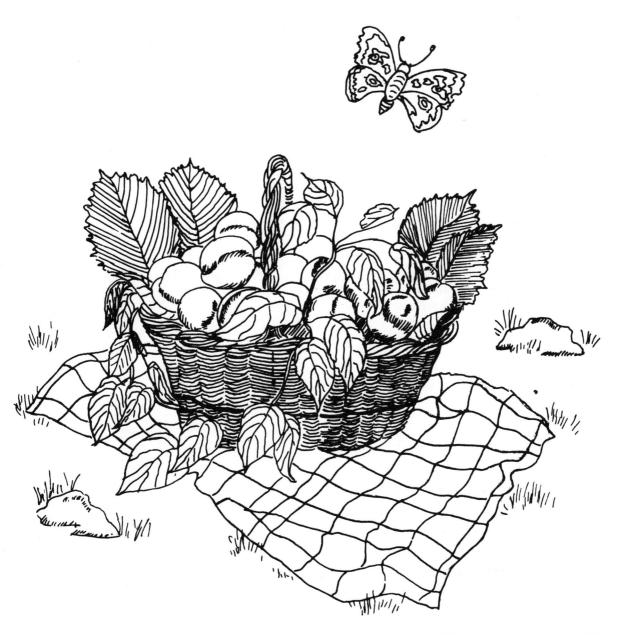

6
For the Sweet Tooth

Apple-Meringue Pie

2 lb apples, cored
2 tbs water or apple cider
4 tbs honey
1 tbs grated lemon rind
2 tsp cinnamon
½ tsp allspice

¼ tsp cloves
1 tbs brandy, optional
3 egg whites
1 tbs honey
pinch of cream of tartar

Peel apples, if desired, cut in half, and slice into thin pieces. Place apples in a skillet with water or cider and honey. Cook over medium heat until apples are barely tender. Stir in lemon rind, cinnamon, allspice, cloves, and brandy. Turn apples into a pie plate or shallow baking dish. Beat egg whites until stiff. Slowly drizzle in honey and cream of tartar and continue beating until honey is well mixed with egg whites. Pile meringue on top of apples, spreading to the edges of the pie plate. Bake in a preheated 275 degree oven for 1 hour, or until meringue is crisp and lightly browned. Serve warm or at room temperature, but do not refrigerate.

Serves 6.

Homemade Cinnamon Applesauce

2 lb apples
½ cup apple cider or water
honey to taste

lemon juice to taste
cinnamon to taste

Core apples and cut into chunks. Place apples and cider or water in a saucepan and simmer until apples are tender. Force mixture through a food mill or

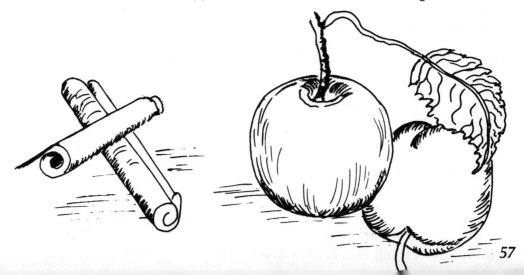

sieve. Season to taste with honey, lemon juice, and cinnamon. The amount of sweetening will vary each time, depending on the sweetness of the apples. To make chunky applesauce, apples must be peeled, seeded, and cut into small cubes before cooking. Simmer apples until tender, then force only a portion of the apples through the food mill, leaving some of the apples in chunks. Serve warm or cold. Makes 3–4 cups.

Apricot-Orange Crêpes Flambé

Crêpe Batter

3 eggs	1 tbs melted butter
1½ cups milk	pinch of sea salt
1 cup whole wheat pastry flour	2 tsp honey
	1 tsp vanilla

Apricot-Orange Sauce

1 pound apricot halves, packed in water or grape juice (available in the diet section of supermarket)	1 cup fresh orange juice
	1 tbs grated orange rind
	½ tsp cornstarch
	¼ cup brandy

Crepe Batter: Place all ingredients in blender and blend until smooth. If necessary, stop blender and scrape down sides. Refrigerate batter for 2 hours before using. Heat a crêpe pan over medium-high heat. Rub pan with a buttered paper towel. Hold pan off the heat and pour a scant ¼ cup batter into pan. Rotate pan quickly so batter covers the bottom, then pour excess batter back into container. Return pan to heat and cook until bottom is lightly browned. Turn crêpe over and cook second side until bottom is dry. Flip crêpe out onto a clean, dry surface. Repeat with remaining batter, lightly buttering the pan only if crêpes begin to stick. This recipe will make 2 dozen crêpes. Extra crêpes may be frozen.

Apricot-Orange Sauce: Cut 8 apricot halves into thin slices and set aside. Place remaining apricots and juice, orange juice, orange rind, and cornstarch in blender. Blend until smooth. Pour into a skillet and cook until slightly thickened. Fold 8 cooked crêpes into quarters. Dip crêpes into sauce, one at a time. Place crêpes

on a heated serving platter and sprinkle with sliced apricots. Pour sauce over crêpes. Warm brandy in a small saucepan. Ignite brandy and pour over crêpes. Serve hot and flaming.
Serves 4.

Honey-Broiled Grapefruit

2 whole grapefruits	cinnamon
2 tbs honey	4 large strawberries

Cut grapefruit in halves; section and use scissors to cut out inner core. Drizzle honey over the surface and sprinkle with cinnamon. Broil grapefruit 2 inches from heat until lightly browned. Place a strawberry in the center of each half and serve warm.
Serves 4.

Rainbow Melon

1 ripe cantaloupe	¼ cup dry white wine, optional
1¾ cups fresh orange juice	honey to taste, optional
1 tbs unflavored gelatin	

Cut melon in half and scoop out seeds. Carefully scrape out a little of the cantaloupe pulp to enlarge the hole in the center. (The extra pulp will make a nice snack.) Soften gelatin in ½ cup orange juice. Place over boiling

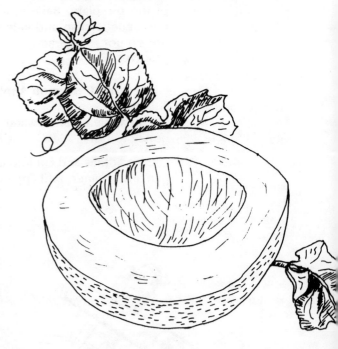

water and stir until gelatin is dissolved. Mix gelatin with remaining orange juice, white wine, and honey to taste. If the oranges are sweet, no honey will be needed. If not using white wine, add ¼ cup more orange juice. Pour mixture into cantaloupe halves and refrigerate until set. Any extra gelatin may be poured into a separate bowl. Carefully cut cantaloupe into halves. Serve on individual plates on a bed of shiny green leaves.

Variation: This dessert is lovely when made with honeydew melon and raspberry gelatin. To make the gelatin, purée enough fresh raspberries in the blender to make two cups of juice. Strain. Follow recipe above, omitting white wine. If melons are large, cut each half into three sections, after gelatin has set, to make six servings.

Lemon Mousse in Orange Shells

2 tbs unflavored gelatin	4 egg yolks
⅓ cup cold water	2 tsp grated lemon rind
⅓ cup honey	1 tbs Marsala, optional
2 tbs lemon juice	6 egg whites
1⅓ cups water	6 oranges

Soften gelatin in ⅓ cup cold water. Place honey, lemon juice, and 1⅓ cups water in the top of a double boiler over hot water. When mixture is hot, beat in egg yolks, one at a time. Continue cooking, stirring constantly, until mixture is thickened. Stir in gelatin, lemon rind, and Marsala. Cook until gelatin is dissolved. Pour into a bowl and set aside until mixture cools. Beat egg whites until stiff. Fold whites into lemon mixture. Cut tops off oranges and use a sharp knife to scoop out all the pulp. Reserve pulp for another use. Dry orange shells with a paper towel. Pile lemon mousse into orange shells and refrigerate until well chilled. Garnish with fresh mint leaves and serve on a bed of shiny green leaves. Note: If you prefer not to use the orange shells, pour lemon mousse into a souffle dish and refrigerate until set.

Serves 6.

Spicy Poached Pears

½ cup orange juice	1 cinnamon stick,
½ cup red wine	broken in half
2 slivers lemon rind	6 whole cloves
2 slivers orange rind	4 whole pears
1 tbs honey	

Place all ingredients, except pears, in a small saucepan and bring to a boil. Peel pears, cut in half, and remove cores. Place pears in saucepan and simmer for 10 minutes, or until barely tender. Spoon sauce over pears several times while cooking. With a slotted spoon, remove pears to a serving dish. Boil remaining sauce for 2 minutes. Strain sauce and pour over pears. Serve warm or refrigerate until well chilled.

Serves 4.

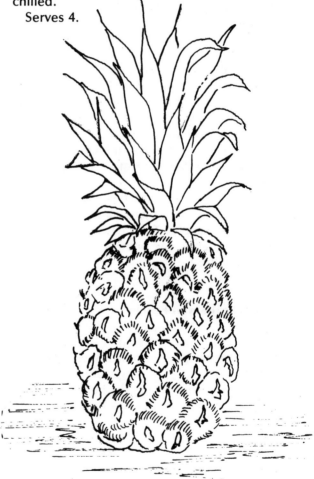

Pineapple Upside-Down Cake

¼ cup honey	⅓ cup honey
1 tbs butter	1 tbs safflower oil
2 tbs chopped pecans or walnuts	4 tbs water
	1 tsp vanilla

1 8-oz can
 unsweetened
 pineapple slices,
 drained
2 eggs, separated

1 cup whole wheat
 pastry flour
1½ tsp baking powder
pinch of sea salt

Place ¼ cup honey and 1 tbs butter in a saucepan and heat just until butter melts. Pour this into the bottom of an 8-inch square shallow baking dish. Sprinkle with nuts. Cut each pineapple slice into 6 pieces. Arrange pineapple in a single layer over the honey-butter mixture. Place egg yolks, honey, and oil in a bowl. Beat by hand or with an electric mixer until light and creamy. Stir in water and vanilla. Sift together the flour, baking powder, and salt. Stir flour mixture into egg yolk mixture. In a separate bowl, beat egg whites until stiff. Gently fold whites into batter. Carefully pour batter over pineapple. Bake in a preheated 350 degree oven for 30 to 35 minutes, or until a toothpick inserted in the center comes out clean. Let cool for 10 minutes. Run a knife around edges of the cake, then invert it onto a serving platter. Serve warm or at room temperature.

Variation: Sliced peaches, apricot halves, cherries, or sliced apples may be substituted for the pineapple. Two teaspoons cinnamon may be added to the honey-butter glaze for a spicy topping.
Serves 10.

Puff Pancake with Peaches

Batter

3 eggs, separated
⅓ cup milk
3 tbs whole wheat
 pastry flour

pinch of sea salt
2 tsp vanilla
1½ tbs honey
1½ tbs butter

Peaches

1 lb peaches
2 tbs honey
3 tbs white wine,
 water, or orange
 juice

1 tsp cinnamon

Batter: Place egg yolks, milk, flour, salt, vanilla, and 1½ tbs honey in a bowl and mix well. In a separate bowl, beat egg whites until stiff.

Fold whites into yolk mixture. Heat butter in a 10-inch ovenproof skillet. When butter is sizzling, pour batter into skillet. Bake in a preheated 400 degree oven for 8 to 10 minutes, or until set. Place on a serving platter and cover with sautéed peaches. Serve at once.

To prepare peaches: Peel and slice peaches. Place them in a skillet with 2 tbs honey and wine, water, or orange juice. Sauté peaches until barely tender. Stir in cinnamon. Peaches should be served warm.

Variation: Serve Puff Pancake with sautéed apples or applesauce instead of the peaches.
Serves 4.

Strawberry Delight

1 tbs unflavored
 gelatin
⅓ cup cold water
1 pt strawberries
1 tsp lemon juice

2 to 3 tbs honey to
 taste
3 egg whites

Soften gelatin in cold water. Place over boiling water and stir until gelatin is dissolved. Place gelatin and all remaining ingredients, except egg whites, in blender. Blend until very smooth. Pour into a bowl and refrigerate until thickened, but not set. Beat egg whites until stiff. Fold whites into strawberry mixture. Pour into individual wine glasses and refrigerate until set and well chilled. If desired, garnish with sliced fresh strawberries and a few mint leaves.
Serves 4.

Watermelon Boat with Fresh Fruit Compote

½ watermelon, cut
 lengthwise
1 cantaloupe
½ lb seedless green
 grapes
4 peaches

½ fresh pineapple
1 pt strawberries
3 tbs honey
juice of 2 oranges
1 tsp lemon juice
½ cup chopped dates

Remove watermelon from its shell; seed and cut into small cubes. If desired, the edge of the watermelon shell may be scalloped or cut into a zig-zag pattern. Remove seeds and rind from cantaloupe and cut into cubes. Peel and slice peaches. Cut pineapple into cubes. Mix all ingredients together and refrigerate, covered, until serving time. Pour fruit compote into

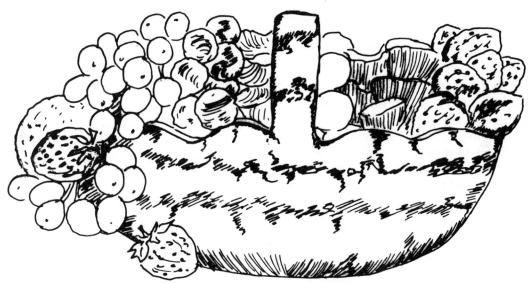

watermelon shell and garnish with fresh mint leaves.

Serves 12.

Yogurt Fruit Parfait

1 tbs unflavored gelatin	1 cup unsweetened crushed pineapple, drained
¼ cup cold water	1 cup sliced strawberries
3 tbs honey	
2 cups plain yogurt	
1 tsp vanilla	4 whole strawberries

Soften gelatin in cold water. Place over boiling water and stir until gelatin is dissolved. Gently mix gelatin with honey, yogurt, vanilla, pineapple, and sliced strawberries. Pour mixture into 4 parfait or wine glasses and refrigerate until set and well chilled. Garnish with whole strawberries before serving.

Serves 4.

Frozen Vanilla Yogurt

1 tbs unflavored gelatin	⅓ to ½ cup honey to taste
¼ cup cold water	⅓ cup powdered milk
¼ cup boiling water	1 tbs vanilla
3 cups plain yogurt	

Soften gelatin in cold water. Add boiling water and stir until gelatin is dissolved. Place gelatin and all remaining ingredients in blender and blend until smooth. Pour mixture into an ice-cream freezer and churn-freeze. *Or*, pour mixture into a bowl and place in the freezer for 2 to 3 hours, until partially frozen. Remove from freezer and beat with an electric mixer until smooth. Serve at once, for soft-frozen yogurt. Or cover and return to freezer and let soften at room temperature 15 minutes before serving.

Frozen Fruit Yogurt: Add 1½ cups fresh fruit to the yogurt before blending. Experiment with different fruits until you find your own favorite: strawberries, raspberries (should be puréed first, then strained), peaches, blueberries, bananas, apricots, prunes, canned unsweetened pineapple.

Serves 6.

Pineapple-Buttermilk Sherbet

1 tbs unflavored gelatin	2 cups buttermilk
¼ cup cold water	¼ cup honey
¼ cup boiling water	2 tsp vanilla
1 20-oz can unsweetened crushed pineapple	

Soften gelatin in cold water. Add boiling water and stir until gelatin is dissolved. Place all ingredients, including gelatin, in blender. Blend until smooth. Pour into a bowl and freeze until mixture is partially frozen. Beat with an electric mixer until smooth. Pour into freezer container, cover, and return to freezer. Let soften at room temperature 15 minutes before serving.

Serves 6 to 8.

Strawberry Ice

2 pints strawberries, hulled
1/3 cup honey
1/2 cup water
1 tbs brandy or 2 tsp lemon juice

Place all ingredients in blender and blend until smooth. Pour into a bowl and place in freezer. When partially frozen, remove from freezer and beat with an electric mixer until smooth. Serve at once or pour into a freezer container, cover tightly, and freeze. Let soften at room temperature 15 minutes before serving.

For a special dessert, serve Strawberry Ice in fresh, peeled peach halves, allowing two halves per person. Garnish with fresh mint leaves. It is also lovely served in hollowed-out lemon shells.

Sunshine Sherbet

1 tbs unflavored gelatin
1/4 cup cold water
1/4 cup boiling water
3 cups fresh orange juice
2 tbs lemon juice
3 bananas
1/2 cup nonfat powdered milk
2 tsp vanilla
honey to taste, optional
2 egg whites

Soften gelatin in cold water. Add boiling water and stir until gelatin is dissolved. In two batches, place all ingredients, except egg whites, in blender and blend until very smooth. Pour into a bowl. In a separate bowl, beat egg whites until stiff. Fold into orange mixture. Freeze until partially frozen, then beat with an electric mixer until smooth. Pour into a container, cover tightly, and freeze. Let soften at room temperature 15 minutes before serving.

Note: This is beautiful served in hollowed-out orange shells, placed on a bed of green leaves, and garnished with a ring of fresh daisies. Makes 6 cups.

Ginger Snaps

5 tbs butter
5 tbs honey
1/4 cup molasses
1 1/2 cups whole wheat pastry flour
1/8 tsp baking soda
1/8 tsp sea salt
3 tsp ginger
1/2 tsp cinnamon

Using an electric mixer, cream together the butter, honey, and molasses until light and fluffy. Stir in all remaining ingredients. Dough will be sticky, but knead until it holds together.

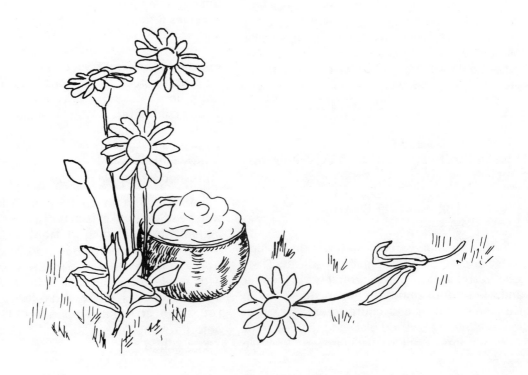

Flatten into a large pancake and place in the freezer for 10 to 15 minutes. Remove dough from freezer and knead dough until smooth. Roll dough out as thin as possible on a floured board. Cut into rounds with a cookie cutter (one with scalloped edges is especially nice), and place on an ungreased cookie sheet. Bake in a preheated 350 degree oven for 8 minutes, or until lightly browned. Cool on a wire rack, then store in an airtight container.

Makes 3 dozen cookies.

Lemon Crisps

5 tbs butter	1½ cups whole wheat
⅓ cup honey	pastry flour
1 heaping tbs grated	⅛ tsp baking soda
lemon rind	⅛ tsp sea salt
1 tsp vanilla	

Follow directions for making Ginger Snaps as appropriate, but substitute the ingredients listed above.

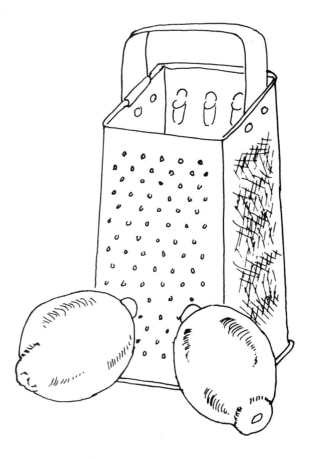

7
Start the Day Right

Yogurt Sundae

¾ cup plain yogurt
1 tsp to 1 tbs honey to taste
1 tbs sunflower seeds
½ tbs sesame seeds
1 tbs slivered almonds

1 tbs raisins
⅓ cup fresh fruit of your
    choice—sliced banana,
    blueberries, strawberries,
    peaches, etc.

Place yogurt in a serving bowl and mix with honey. Top with seeds, nuts, raisins, and fresh fruit.

Variation: Stir in 1 tbs unprocessed bran.

Note: The seeds, nuts, and raisins may be mixed together in large quantities and stored in a jar. Use 1 part sesame seeds and 2 parts sunflower seeds, almonds, and raisins. One part cashews and/or pumpkin seeds may be added if desired.

Serves 1.

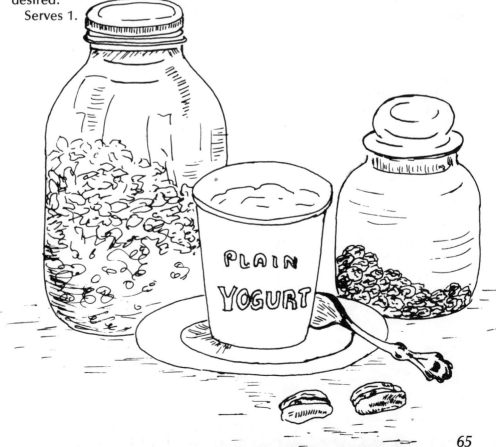

Yogurt and Fruit Smoothie

1 cup plain yogurt	1 small banana
1 tsp to 1 tbs honey to taste	½ tsp vanilla
	3 to 4 ice cubes

Place all ingredients in the blender and blend until smooth. For additional protein, add 1 raw egg before blending.

Variation: 1 tbs frozen orange juice concentrate or ½ cup fresh fruit may be added to the smoothie. Peaches, nectarines, pineapple or strawberries are great, too.

Serves 1.

Herb Omelet

3 eggs	¼ tsp tarragon, dill, or basil
2 tbs cold water	
pinch of sea salt	1 tbs parsley, chopped
2 tsp butter	
2 tsp chives, chopped	

Place eggs, water, and salt in a small bowl and whisk together until foamy. Melt butter in an omelet pan. When butter sizzles, pour in eggs. Cook over medium-high heat, and use a spatula to lift around the edges to let liquid eggs run underneath. When omelet is almost set—soft on top but firm on the bottom—sprinkle on the chives, herbs, and parsley. When omelet is set, fold in half and serve.

Variations: *Cheese Omelet*—add 3 tbs cottage cheese or grated Cheddar cheese at the same time as the herbs. *Sprout Omelet*—mix 1 tsp tamari with the eggs. Add 3 tbs alfalfa sprouts with the herbs.

Serves 2.

Spanish Omelet

1 tbs safflower oil	½ tsp thyme or marjoram
1 onion, chopped	
1 celery stalk, chopped	herb salt and pepper to taste
1 green pepper, chopped	3 eggs
2 tomatoes, peeled	2 tbs water
	pinch of sea salt
1 tbs parsley, chopped	2 tsp butter

Heat oil in a skillet and sauté onion, celery, and green pepper for 5 minutes. Cut peeled tomatoes in half and gently squeeze out seeds and excess liquid. Chop into small pieces. Add tomatoes, parsley, thyme or marjoram, herb salt, and pepper to the pan. Simmer for 8 minutes, or until mixture is almost dry. Whisk eggs, water, and sea salt together. Melt butter in an omelet pan and cook eggs as directed in previous recipe. When omelet is almost set, spoon 3 tbs vegetables over the eggs. Fold omelet in half and serve. Any extra sauce may be used for additional omelets; or refrigerate it, then reheat when needed.

Baked Puffy Omelet

3 eggs, separated	¼ tsp tarragon or dill, optional
¼ cup cottage cheese	
1 tbs onion, minced, optional	herb salt and pepper to taste
1 tbs parsley, chopped	1 tbs butter

Place egg yolks, cottage cheese, onion, parsley, tarragon, herb salt, and pepper in a bowl and whisk together until fluffy. Beat egg whites in a separate bowl until stiff. Fold whites into beaten yolks. Melt butter until it sizzles in an 8-inch ovenproof skillet. Pour in eggs and cook over low heat until omelet begins to rise. Place in a preheated 375 degree oven for 10 to 15 minutes, or until omelet is puffy and slightly browned. Cut into wedges and serve at once.

Serves 2.

Egg Foo Yung

Batter

4 eggs	1 tbs parsley, chopped
1 celery stalk, minced	1 cup bean sprouts
1 to 2 scallions, minced	sea salt to taste
	safflower oil

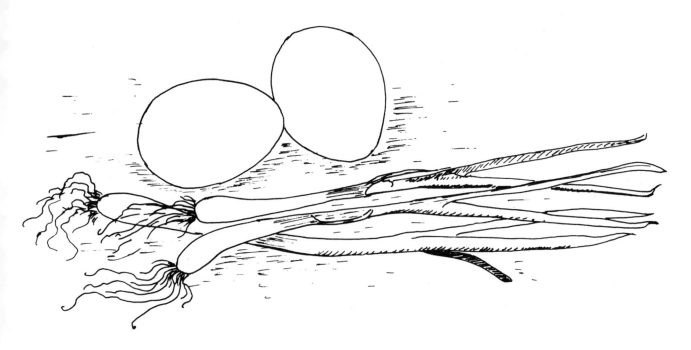

Sauce

¾ cup chicken broth   1½ tbs cornstarch *or*
  or vegetable broth   arrowroot
1 tbs soy sauce   2 tbs water

Place eggs in a bowl and whisk until foamy. Stir in all remaining ingredients, except oil. Place a small amount of oil in a skillet and rub with a paper towel so the oil coats the entire pan. When the skillet is quite hot, drop batter into the pan by tablespoons. When bottom is lightly browned, flip pancake over with a spatula and brown the second side. Use additional oil to cook the rest of the batter. Serve at once with the following sauce.

Sauce: Heat broth and soy sauce in a small saucepan. Mix cornstarch or arrowroot with water to form a paste and stir into broth. Cook just until sauce is slightly thickened. Spoon hot sauce over egg foo yung.
Serves 2.

Creamy Cottage Cheese Pancakes

1½ cups low-fat   ¼ tsp sea salt
  cottage cheese   juice of half an orange
4 large eggs   3 tsp baking powder
2 tbs safflower oil   ¾ cup whole wheat
1 tsp honey   pastry flour

Place all ingredients in a bowl and whisk together. Place a small amount of oil in a skillet—just enough so the pancakes won't stick—and heat to medium-high. Drop batter into skillet by the spoonful and cook until brown on the bottom. Flip pancakes and cook just until browned. Serve with blueberry sauce, applesauce, or sliced fresh fruit and yogurt.
Serves 4.

Buttermilk Waffles

1½ cups buttermilk   ½ tsp. sea salt
4 eggs, separated   2 tbs safflower oil
1½ cups whole wheat 1 tbs baking powder
  pastry flour   2 tsp vanilla

Place buttermilk and egg yolks in a bowl and beat with a whisk until foamy. Add remaining ingredients, except egg whites, and stir until batter is smooth. Beat egg whites until stiff. Fold egg whites into batter. Bake in a hot waffle iron until done. Serve with blueberry sauce.
Serves 4.

Strawberry-Cheese Sandwich

1 slice whole grain   cinnamon
  bread   ½ cup strawberries
2 oz farmer's cheese ½ tsp vanilla

Place bread in toaster and toast slightly. Spread toast with farmer's cheese and sprinkle with cinnamon. Broil until cheese is puffed and lightly browned. Crush strawberries with a fork and mix with vanilla. Top broiled sandwich with crushed strawberries and serve at once. Serves 1.

Raisin Bran Muffins

1 cup unprocessed
  bran
1 cup plus 1 tbs
  buttermilk
1 egg, beaten
¼ cup honey
2 tbs safflower oil

1 tsp vanilla
1¼ cups whole wheat
  pastry flour
2 tsp baking powder
½ tsp sea salt
½ cup raisins

Soak bran in buttermilk for 15 minutes. Stir in beaten egg, honey, oil, and vanilla. Mix well. Sift together the flour, baking powder, and salt. Gently stir flour and raisins into bran mixture—batter will be slightly lumpy. Pour batter into buttered muffin tins. Bake in a preheated 375 degree oven for 20 to 25 minutes. Muffins are done when a toothpick inserted in the center comes out clean. Muffins may be frozen, then reheated in a 350 degree oven for 10 to 15 minutes. Makes 1 dozen.

Whole Wheat Bread

2¼ cups warm water
  (105 degrees to 115
  degrees)

¾ cup powdered milk
⅓ cup safflower oil
2 tsp sea salt

2 tbs active dry yeast
⅓ cup honey
6 to 7 cups
  stoneground whole
  wheat flour

2 eggs, beaten, at
  room temperature

In a large mixing bowl, dissolve yeast and 1 tbs honey in warm water. Let stand 5 to 10 minutes, until foamy. Stir in 2¼ cups whole wheat flour. Beat 100 strokes by hand or 3 to 4 minutes with an electric mixer. Cover bowl with a towel and allow sponge to rise in a warm place until doubled in bulk, about 45 minutes. Stir in remaining honey, powdered milk, oil, salt, eggs, and 4 cups flour. Turn out onto a well-floured board and knead thoroughly for 8 to 10 minutes, until dough is smooth and elastic. (This takes a lot of muscle, but it's good exercise for your arms.) Add only enough additional flour as necessary to keep dough from sticking to the board. Place dough in a large oiled bowl, turn once to oil top of dough. Cover with a damp towel and set in a warm place, about 75 to 80 degrees. Let rise until doubled in bulk.

Punch down dough, and divide in half. Roll each half into a rectangle, approximately 9 by 14 inches. Starting at one short end, roll dough tightly. Pinch to seal ends and turn under. Place seam side down in two 9-by-5-by-3-inch buttered loaf pans. Cover and put in a warm place until dough reaches the top of the pan. Bake in a preheated 350 degree oven for 50 to

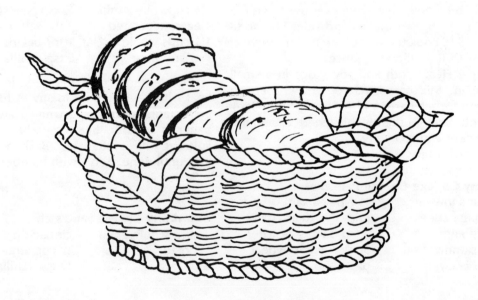

60 minutes. To test if bread is done, tap the crust to see if it makes a hollow sound. Remove from pans and brush top of bread with butter. Cool on wire racks. Bread may be frozen when it is cool. Makes 2 loaves.

See the following variations:

Sprouted Wheat Bread. Substitute 2 cups sprouted wheat berries for 2 cups of whole wheat flour.

Cracked Wheat Bread. Add ½ cup cracked wheat to 1 cup boiling water. Let stand 1 hour. Stir mixture into whole wheat dough.

Oatmeal Bread. Substitute 1¼ cups rolled oats for 1¼ cups of the whole wheat flour mixed into the sponge. Molasses may be substituted for all or part of the honey.

Sunflower Bread. Use ½ cup sunflower seeds or sesame seeds mixed into whole wheat dough.

Lighter Wheat Bread. Unbleached white flour may be substituted for up to one-half the amount of whole wheat flour called for. The resulting bread will be lighter and easier to knead, but not as nutritious. If this is your first attempt at making bread, this is a good dough to start with.

Raisin Bread. Knead 1½ cups raisins into the dough before the first rising. For cinnamon bread, mix 2 tbs cinnamon with the other ingredients before kneading.

Dutch Apple Oatmeal

1¼ cups rolled oats	2½ tbs honey
1½ cups low-fat milk	1 tsp vanilla
1¼ cups water	½ tsp cinnamon
¼ tsp sea salt	
1 to 2 apples, cored, grated, or cut in tiny cubes	

Place oats, milk, water, and salt in a saucepan and let stand 10 minutes. Bring to a boil. Reduce heat and simmer 10 to 15 minutes, until oatmeal is thick and creamy. Stir in apples, honey, vanilla, and cinnamon. Serve hot.

Serves 4.

Swiss Muesli

3 tbs rolled oats	honey to taste
⅓ cup water	1 tsp lemon juice
2 tbs milk or yogurt	1 unpeeled apple, grated

Soak rolled oats in water overnight. In the morning, add milk or yogurt, grated apple, honey, and lemon juice.

Variation: When mixing in the apple, add 1 tbs of any of the following—raisins, sunflower seeds, sesame seeds, wheat germ, bran flakes, slivered almonds, fresh fruit, or berries.

Serves 1.

Blueberry Sauce

2 cups blueberries	¼ cup water
¼ to ½ cup honey to taste	1 tsp lemon juice
	pinch of cinnamon

Place all ingredients in a saucepan and cook over low heat until blueberries are tender. Purée in blender until sauce is very smooth. Pour into a jar and store in refrigerator. Serve warm or at room temperature over pancakes, waffles, or plain yogurt. Makes 2½ cups.

Variation: Stir 1 cup fresh whole blueberries into sauce before serving.

Note: If fresh blueberries are not available, substitute frozen, dry-packed blueberries. If a thicker sauce is desired, omit the water.

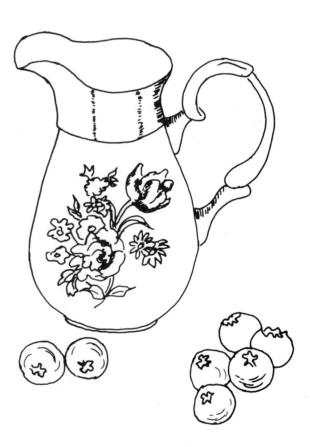

Apple Butter

apples
apple cider or water
honey (very little is needed because apples are naturally sweet)

cinnamon to taste
pinch of ginger, cloves and allspice

Core apples and cut into chunks, leaving peels on. Place in a saucepan with just enough apple cider or water to cover the bottom of the pan. Cover and cook over low heat, stirring occasionally, until apples are very tender. Press apples through a sieve and return to saucepan. Add honey, cinnamon, and other spices to taste. Cook over low heat, uncovered, until very thick. Stir often to prevent scorching.

Pour hot apple butter into hot, sterilized jars and process for 10 minutes in a boiling water bath. *Or*, pour cool apple butter into containers and store in freezer until needed.

Peach Butter. Substitute fresh, pitted peaches for the apples, and orange juice for the cider. Prepare as directed for Apple Butter.

Serves any amount, according to proportions.

Strawberry Jam

1 tbs unflavored gelatin
¼ cup cold water

3 cups strawberries
3 tbs honey
1 tsp lemon juice

Soften gelatin in cold water. Using a fork, coarsely mash strawberries. Place strawberries, honey, and lemon juice in a saucepan. Bring to a boil. Add gelatin and stir until gelatin is dissolved. Pour into a jar and store in refrigerator.

Makes 1 pint.

Grape Jelly

1 tbs unflavored gelatin
2½ cups unsweetened grape juice

¼ cup honey

Soften gelatin in ¼ cup grape juice. Place remaining grape juice in a saucepan and bring to a boil. Add gelatin and honey and stir until gelatin is dissolved. Pour into jars and store in refrigerator. Makes 2¾ cups

Hot, Creamy Carob Drink

2 tbs carob powder
1 tbs honey
1 cup water
¼ cup powdered milk
½ tsp cornstarch *or* arrowroot

pinch of sea salt
pinch of cinnamon
½ tsp vanilla

Place all ingredients, except vanilla, in blender and blend until smooth. Pour into a saucepan and cook over low heat, stirring occasionally, until hot. Stir in vanilla. Pour into a mug and serve at once.

Serves 1.

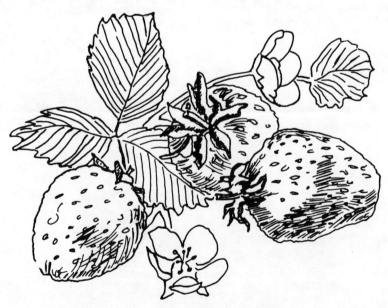

Herb Tea

Whether you want a quick pick up, a soothing tonic for your nerves or digestion, or something to take the edge off your appetite, herb teas are like a little bit of magic in a cup. Herb teas contain no harmful caffeine or tannin, which is found in coffee and black teas. There is an herb tea, with its own unique flavor, to suit every taste and mood. The best way to find out what pleases you is to try a wide variety and then choose your favorites.

Try peppermint tea for breakfast and camomile after dinner. Other popular favorites include rose hip, lemon balm, lemon verbena, papaya, linden, hibiscus, strawberry leaves, and orange blossoms. There are many delightful blends of different herbs available in health food stores.

To prepare herb tea, use one heaping teaspoon of the herb for each cup of water. Place the herb in a stainless steel "tea ball" in a cup or teapot. Pour boiling water over the herbs and let steep for five to ten minutes. Remove tea ball. Taste before sweetening and, if desired, stir in a little honey.

To make iced tea, use 1 tablespoon of herbs per cup of water. Pour boiling water over herbs and let stand until cool. If sweetening is desired, stir in honey before tea cools. Remove tea ball, pour into a bottle, and refrigerate. To serve, pour tea into tall glasses filled with ice. A sprig of fresh mint makes a nice garnish.

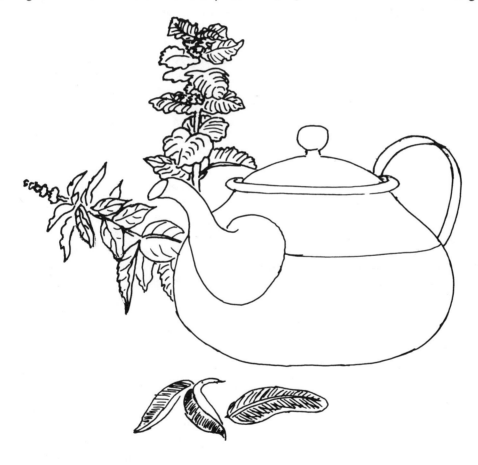

Glossary of Natural Ingredients

Arrowroot A fine, white powder that is made from the roots of the arrowroot plant. It is used as a natural thickening agent and may be substituted for cornstarch.

Baking Powder Always choose aluminum-free low-sodium brands.

Bronner's Broth A salty, natural liquid seasoning made from soybeans and minerals. Complete name to look for is Dr. Bronner's All-One Balanced-Soya-Mineral-Boullion.

Carob Carob powder is made from the dried pods of the carob tree. When ground and roasted, carob has a similar taste and appearance to cocoa and may be used as a substitute for chocolate. Carob is high in natural sugars, vitamins, and minerals. It is low in fat and contains less than half the calories of chocolate.

Herb Salt A natural seasoning made from dried vegetables, herbs, sea salt, and kelp. HerbaMare is an excellent brand.

Honey Use raw, unfiltered honey.

Pita bread A flat, hollow round of bread made from whole wheat or rye flour. Also known as Syrian bread.

Powdered milk Use noninstant, nonfat powdered milk, which has been dried at low temperatures in order to retain the nutritional content of the milk.

Sea Salt Salt containing an abundance of minerals and trace elements, which is made from dried sea water.

Soy Sauce Use soy sauce made from soybeans, wheat, and salt, without sugar and preservatives. A natural soy sauce, with a reduced percentage of salt, is available at "health food" and gourmet shops.

Sprouts Germinating (growing) seeds, beans, or legumes that are extremely low in calories and high in proteins, vitamins, and minerals.

Tahini A smooth, creamy butter made from finely ground sesame seeds. If the sesame butter and oil separate on standing, stir together before using.

Tamari A fermented soy sauce made from soybeans, wheat, and salt, without chemicals and preservatives. If water retention is a problem, use tamari very sparingly, as it is extremely salty.

Tofu Soybean curd, with a firm, custardlike consistency, which is made from fermented soy milk. It is usually found in 2½-inch square pads. The taste is quite bland, but tofu absorbs the flavors of other ingredients it is cooked with. It is a valuable source of protein and unsaturated fats. One 8-ounce serving contains only 147 calories. Store tofu, immersed in a container of water, in the refrigerator.

Wine Wine is optional in many of the recipes, but it does impart a very special flavor to the cooked foods. All of the alcohol and eighty-five percent of the calories are burned off while cooking.

Whole Wheat Pastry Flour Whole wheat flour made from soft winter wheat. May be used for all-purpose baking, to replace white flour, with the exception of yeast breads, which require whole wheat flour because of its higher gluten content.

Suggested Reading

Airola, Paavo, Ph.D., N.D. *Are You Confused?* Phoenix: Health Plus, 1971.

Clark, Linda A. *Be Slim and Healthy*. New Canaan: Keats, 1975.

Clark, Linda A. *Stay Young Longer*. New York: Pyramid Books, 1968.

Davis, Adelle. *Let's Eat Right to Keep Fit*. New York: New American Library, 1970.

Davis, Adelle. *Let's Get Well*. New York: New American Library, 1965.

Deal, Sheldon C., M.D. *New Life Through Nutrition*. Tucson: New Life Publishing, 1974.

Dinaburg, Kathy, and Akel, D'Ann. *Nutrition Survival Kit*. Panjandrum Press, 1976.

Dufty, William. *Sugar Blues*. New York: Warner Books, 1975.

Elwood, Catharyn. *Feel Like a Million*. New York: Pocket Books, 1970.

Fredericks, Carlton, Ph.D. *Carlton Fredericks' Calorie and Carbohydrate Guide*. New York: Pocket Books, 1977.

Fredericks, Carlton, Ph.D. *Dr. Carlton Fredericks' Eat-More-To-Lose-More Diet Book*. Universal Publishing and Distributing Company, 1968.

Fredericks, Carlton, Ph.D. *Dr. Carlton Fredericks' New and Complete Nutrition Book*. Major Books, 1976.

Fredericks, Carlton, Ph.D. and Bailey, Henry. *Food Facts and Fallacies*. New York: Arc Books, 1965.

Fredericks, Carlton, Ph.D. *Look Younger, Feel Healthier*. New York: Grosset & Dunlap, 1975.

Fredericks, Carlton, Ph.D. *Low Blood Sugar and You*. New York: Grosset & Dunlap. 1976.

Goldbeck, Nikki and David. *The Dieter's Companion: A Guide to Nutritional Self-Sufficiency*. New York: New American Library, 1975.

Goldbeck, Nikki and David. *The Supermarket Handbook*. New York: New American Library, 1976.

Hauser, Gayelord. *New Treasury of Secrets*. Greenwich: Fawcett, 1976.

Hunter, Beatrice Trum. *Consumer Beware: Your Food and What's Been Done to It*. New York: Simon and Schuster, 1972.

Hunter, Beatrice Trum. *Fact Book on Food Additives and Your Health*. New Canaan: Keats, 1972.

Hunter, Beatrice Trum. *Natural Foods Primer*. New York: Simon and Schuster, 1972.

Keyes, Ken Jr. *Loving Your Body*. Living Love Center, 1974.

Lappé, Frances Moore, and Collins, Joseph. *Diet for a Small Planet, rev. ed. New York:* Ballantine, 1975.

Passwater, Richard A., Ph.D. *Supernutrition: Megavitamin Revolution*. New York: Pocket Books, 1975.

Watt, Bernice K. and Merrill, Annabel L. *Composition of Foods*. Washington, D.C.: United States Department of Agriculture, 1963.

Williams, Roger J. *Nutrition Against Disease*. New York: Bantam Books, 1973.

Williams, Roger J. *Nutrition in a Nutshell*. New York: Doubleday, 1962.

Williams, Roger J. *The Wonderful World Within You*. New York: Bantam Books, 1977.

Index of Recipes